CAILAH BROCK

DESIGN YOUR BODY

Your Guide To Cutting Through The Fat

ISBN: 978-1-4834-2005-9 (sc)
ISBN: 978-1-4834-2004-2 (e)

Contact Cailah Health Coach Brock:
Email: mss.brock@yahoo.com
Website: www.CailahHealthCoachBrock.com

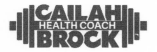

Lulu Publishing Services rev. date: 10/28/2014

CONTENTS

FOREWORD

Congratulations for taking initiative to gain control of your life, mind and body, and preserving your health for years to come. If you are ready to make the commitment to leading a healthy lifestyle, this book will empower you to enhance your quality of life and to attain the healthy mind and body that you deserve.

Cailah Health Coach Brock brings a unique and incredibly realistic approach to healthy living that will yield long-term success for weight loss, weight management, and designing the body of your dreams. While possessing a master's of science in Coaching Education, concentration in Exercise Physiology, from Ohio University and a bachelor's of science in Exercise Science and Fitness Management from the University of Dayton, Cailah is a true fitness enthusiast and professional who leads by example. Through years as a collegiate athlete, coach, personal trainer, fitness instructor, fitness model, and business owner, she has been an advocate for health and fitness her entire life.

This book provides a wealth of information grounded in science and supported by empirical evidence, but more importantly, teaches how to cut through life's many challenges with self-control and positive attitude. While we can't change genetic factors or predispositions to disease, we do have the power to make healthy decisions in our daily lives and re-train the mind to think positively. Cailah demonstrates that with a positive attitude, success and results will follow.

If you trust in Cailah's process, you can be the best version of yourself and an inspiration to others. This book is more than a guide to weight management, but a tool to achieving success in all areas of life.

With an open heart and mind to Cailah's guide, you will experience the true meaning of healthy living and unveil the secret to sustainable results.

-Allyson Caudell, MS

PREFACE

In the health and fitness world, there are a multitude of resources that encourage weight loss. Each resource has its own set of guidelines, exercises and patterns of cause and effect that don't always align with science and/or research. Information regarding health and wellness has become muddled, muddied and made-up of gimmicks promoting the best diet, diet pill, shakes, smoothies, gluten free products, protein or even surgery. So how can health seekers expect to know what is real and what will work? Design Your Body: Your Guide to Cutting Through The Fat was written to purify the water and help people have a clear voice and true insight on the steps they need to take in creating and maintaining a journey of weight loss and a venturing into a new lifestyle. Start a new path today. Reinvent yourself and achieve the goals that have become distant dreams.

ACKNOWLEDGMENTS

To those who contributed to the creation of the book: Words cannot express my thankfulness in receiving your prayers, guidance and assistance. A simple "thank you" isn't enough, so I've immortalized your names within this section of love.

Inspirational and Financial Contributors:

- Gayle and Daryl Brock
- Terrence & Yolanda Sherrer
- Stephanie James
- Stephanie Hughes
- Trish Kitchell
- Linda Suggs
- Pietra Foster
- Brittney Johnson
- Knasarae Orr
- Allyson Caudell
- Jesiah Brock

- Jason White, PhD
- Dafina-Lazarus Stewart, PhD
- Cimmon Burris
- Melissa Douglass
- Kay and Charlie Rutherford
- Adrienne Carrington
- Candace Oglesby
- Henry & Lynn Long
- Patricia Corbett - editor
- Lawrence Givens - photographer
- Evan Murray - photographer

"If I inspire you, you are my inspiration"
-Stephanie James bka Just A Vessel

INTRODUCTION

Disclaimer; this is not a book full of warm fuzzies, emotional rises or empty encouragements. This book will provide you with facts and concrete steps towards improving your health. Choose your starting point, and I'll take you the rest of the way.

Almost everyone says they want to lose weight, but the question is, are you ready to commit? Weight loss pills, starving yourself or the diet-of-the-month may seem like a good idea or they may even work for a few weeks but they do not last.

Dieting is not a lifestyle. The very word "diet" indicates a temporary occurrence, which is why those who diet tend to experience fluctuating weight loss. They also typically experience a roller coaster to health. Weight loss pills encourage you to spend money on a product that may momentarily cause weight loss, but you run the extreme risk of malnutrition and other serious health risks as most are not federally regulated. There is also a very real risk of developing a physiological and psychological dependency on these products. Dietary supplements encourage you to become dependent on the product leaving you financially drained, reliant on products rather than food. More importantly, consumers generally still ill-informed about the proper procedures leading to good health.

I am not going to create empty weight loss promises or guarantees because each reader has their own goals and very different starting points. Most importantly, each reader will have different levels of commitment to this program. But I will say that adhering to this guide which is packed full of factual and scientific data can and will allow you to reduce the amount of prescribed medications, reduce High Blood Pressure (hypertension), eliminate Type II Diabetes, lower your risk for other metabolic diseases and of course, initiate weight loss allowing you to maintain a healthy lifestyle.

This guide will assist you in creating your own personal plan for 'designing your body' while gradually changing your lifestyle. Weight loss should not be a temporary fad; but in today's culture, we live in a "microwave society" where we want everything to appear immediately and if things do not quickly unfold, we quit and blame the system. Expecting to lose weight fast is like putting a 20lb turkey in the oven for 30 minutes (which barely raises its' core temperature) and expecting a lavish meal to take the same amount of time as it does to reheat a frozen dinner. I promise you, this will take longer than 2 minutes. It will take more than a day, more than a month and it may take more than a year to reach your goal. Creating a new lifestyle first requires "un-living" the old one. If you are truly ready to lose weight and become a healthier you, then I'll show you how to change your life!

You must be aware that the journey to gaining and maintaining weight loss and better health is long-term. Again, this will not happen overnight, you may not see any changes in your body until month two! But sticking to this guide and the program will help you create, accomplish, and maintain your goal for years to come. I will teach you how to lose weight, keep it off, and shape your body to your liking. If you follow my instructions to the "T" and give me time, effort, and enthusiasm, I will Design Your Body.

DEDICATION

This book is dedicated to those who have decided to change their state of life, and to those who aren't afraid of sweat or hard work. This guide is for all who are actively seeking a better physical life, the millions of Americans who are overweight, and those who are not satisfied with their multiple attempts to lose and maintain weight loss. This journey will not be easy and is a continuous process. Cheers to you for making a decision to move towards improving your quality of life and taking the first step in a lifestyle change that will allow you to Design Your Body! Runners! To your marks!

PART I

Getting Started

CHAPTER 1

Are You Ready to Commit?

Determining whether you are mentally ready to create and <u>maintain</u> change in your life will dictate your potential success in adhering to this program and experiencing lifelong results. When it comes to the thought or idea of change, there are five stages we as humans' experience. These scientifically documented stages are; Precontemplation, Contemplation, Preparation, Action and Maintenance.

The Transtheoretical Model of Change (Prochaska & Marcus, 1994) is a behavioral theory which examines an individual's readiness to change by identifying which of the five stages best represents their current behavioral and mental stance (Bryant & Green, 2011, p. 487). Use these stages to pinpoint your level of readiness.

Precontemplation

Precontemplation is simply that. This is the point before the thought of change has even become an idea or entered your mind. People in this stage may understand that they are overweight or unhealthy, but they have never entertained the thought of acting to become healthy. People in this stage are generally sedentary and are not at the point of considering their need for change. Individuals in this stage do not view their health as an important aspect of their lives and often sneer at the idea of being physically active or taking steps to make healthy changes.

Contemplation

Individuals in this stage are still sedentary although they are beginning to consider the consequences of their current habits and lifestyle. They may have thought about exercise, or becoming healthy, but it's just a thought. These individuals are still not ready for exercise, nor are they prepared to commit or create change. This may be your current position; you are thinking about becoming healthy but either you don't know where to start, or you are not yet serious about the changes that need to occur in your life. If this stage describes you, do me a favor; take a moment to look at your life, health, happiness, habits, family, job and general lifestyle. From a wellness standpoint, where do you see yourself in five years? How will your current lifestyle dictate your future? Is the vision of you five years from now positive? Do you need to change? What can you do to change? What are the steps you need to take? Step 1 – get serious and start planning.

Preparation

In this stage, people have begun to make moves towards their goals of a healthy life and weight loss. They may have walked, exercised, done some research or even bought this book. They have started acting on their ideas and have begun to create and act on a weight loss plan for a few days to weeks. These individuals are mentally, emotionally and physically preparing to adopt a healthier lifestyle. They are in the process of committing to change, though many actions may be inconsistent. You may be in this stage and I encourage you to continue on this path and stay consistent. The only failure in health and wellness is quitting. Be successful in your journey by not stopping, regressing or quitting, no matter how hard, long or grueling your journey may become.

Action

People in this stage are committed to creating a new plan and have already consistently put that plan into motion. They have begun exercising and consistently eating healthy (1 – 6 months). If this is you, keep it up! Do not allow monotony, disappointments, schedules or general difficulties hinder you from continuing on this track. You may or may not experience the weight loss you expected at your 6 month mark but use this guide to push you past the plateau and further into Designing Your Body.

Maintenance

Those who find themselves in this stage have engaged in creating a healthier lifestyle for themselves for over 6 months. This may also be you. Those in this stage may find themselves fighting the plateau. Stay encouraged! Weight loss often occurs in phases and your body adapts to learned habits. Use this resource to assist you in recreating an exercise plan that pushes you past your plateau and to further healthy weight loss.

Depending on which stage best pinpoints your current state, what is your level of commitment? If you find yourself in the Contemplation or Preparation stage, let's get serious about your weight loss journey! No more playing games and no more fooling around. Make a commitment to give the program in this book your best effort possible. Commitment = Success. If you commit yourself to learning more about general health, your body, participating in exercise and improving your nutrition habits, you are bound to succeed! But your success is dependent upon your commitment to the habits we will create. Do not allow yourself to slip from the Action stage to Contemplation, stay consistent, and stick it through knowing you will encounter a roller coaster of emotions, weight gains and losses and feelings of doubt. STICK TO IT because commitment = success. Stick to it and carve out the body that you want and deserve. Just stick to it!

To prove your level of commitment to yourself, to your family and friends, read and complete the below pledge to stay committed to self-preservation, self-improvement and Designing Your Body.

I, _____, pledge to fully commit myself to making better decisions and actions regarding my health, fitness and nutrition to create a more desirable lifestyle for me. I am fully aware that this is a long and slow process and that desirable change will not occur overnight, but I commit myself to becoming my best self through hard work, determination, commitment and diligence. I understand that there are times where I may want to quit, but on this _____ day of _____ in the year _____, I am promising myself that I will do better, I will be better, and I WILL NOT QUIT!

_____   _____
Your Signature   Signature of Witness

"Set your mind on being good, being happy, and being healthy."
-Cailah Brock

It's game time! Here is what you need to be successful

1. Long Term Change

If you're reading this book, you may be aware that your current lifestyle may not be the best way to reach your goals of weight loss. You may also be looking for different or better results than what your current program provides. Many people know and understand their habits are the antithesis of healthy, but they aren't willing to change or amend behaviors while seeking better results. Albert Einstein states that insanity is continually doing the same thing, but seeking different results. It's time for a change.

> *"Insanity: Doing the same thing over and over*
> *again and expecting different results"*
> *-Albert Einstein*

2. Positive and Driven mindset

In certain cultures and tribes in Africa, the people have the thought and belief that a certain look from the Shaman could kill you. There have also been reported cases of individuals on the receiving end of this "look" who have passed away shortly thereafter. Were these people killed by the Shaman's look, or did they mentally commit suicide? This 'Shaman belief' suggests that your mind is the most powerful asset you possess and your thoughts can be detrimental. Your mind drives your actions, responses, interpretations state of mind and state of being on a daily basis.

Imagine yourself reaching the level where you decide to have a good day as opposed to allowing situations to rule your atmosphere. Imagine being able to tell yourself, "No", to soda pop, sugar, cakes, candy and other unnecessary carbs. Imagine being in full control of you! Well, ladies and gentlemen; I am granting you that power. I am granting you the access to fully recruit and command your mind. You are privy to the knowledge that you possess and you have the capacity to control your entire atmosphere. The first step is to will your mind to be successful, happy and healthy. Along your journey to health and good fitness, you must control your mind and will success into each set, each rep and each minute of exercise. Will yourself to win this battle for your life for yourself, your family and those whom you hold dear. Though some days will be easier than others, as long as you will yourself to succeed and make hard decisions that will lead towards a better you, you will not lose the war.

Though mental strength and will is extremely valuable, nothing happens without action.

"Faith without works is dead."
-James 2:17

CHAPTER 2

Setting S.M.A.R.T. Goals

In order to accomplish a task, it is imperative to set goals and benchmarks. Those possessing thoughts, wishes and dreams which lack direction and vision, remain stuck in their dreams. The most effective way of making your aspirations attainable is by setting planned and structured steps leading to full accomplishment. Some individuals are good planners and this chapter will be a breeze in helping you create your goals. For those who struggle with planning and prefer spontaneity, you may have thought that your goal of weight loss is obvious and does not need an explanation. Though this is understandable, it is important to note; those who do not detail their goals and create means to maintain progress typically fail. I encourage you to follow through with these first steps which will create a rock solid foundation to 'Designing Your Body'.

"Where there is no vision, the people perish."
-Proverbs 29:18

Specific:

Goals must be specific. Overarching goals such as "weight loss" does not designate an end result. This goal is extremely broad. If your goal is simply weight loss, well, go use the restroom and you will have accomplished just that.

The below questions should be answered when creating your Specific goal

- Who, besides yourself does this goal involve?

  _____

- What do you want to accomplish?

  _____

- Where should this goal be accomplished?

  _____

- Why/what is the purpose of this goal?

  _____

- What are the constraints to you reaching this goal?

  _____

In writing your specific goal, also note; this goal can be objective or subjective. Objective goals involve physically tangible facts or results often including hard data such as numbers, titles, or other verifiable data.

Example; "I want to lose 30lbs", "I want to increase my paycheck from $2,000/month to $3,000/month", "I want to improve my free-throw shooting percentage to 80%", "I want to become an Executive Director at my job", "I want to earn a graduate degree" etc. Notice how each of these goals are concrete, specific and based on hard data or fact.

Subjective goals are goals that are not entirely based upon fact or hard data, but are more driven by opinion and personal feelings.

Example; "I want to be prettier", "I want to be happier with my body", "I want more people to like me", "I want to be healthier", "I want a better sex life" etc.

Knowing your current weight status is imperative. Your total weight isn't just one number, it is a figure that comprises four different variables: Protein (muscles), minerals (bone), water and fats (essential and nonessential). Breaking this down into more digestible portions; your body is more easily categorized as Fat Free Mass (FFM) or Fat Mass (FM). Fat Free Mass includes muscle, bone and water while and

FM is pure fat. When looking at your scale, it may read 246lbs. This total number should not indicate life or death in your mind as this figure only represents total mass. You should be focused on the composition of your total mass.

Understanding what your Body Composition is will help you set attainable and realistic goals. For example; if you weigh 246lbs and 34% of you is FM while 66% of you is FFM. Thirty four percent of 246lbs = 83.64lbs of FM, allowing you to set a specific goal of losing 50lbs (notice how the weight loss goal is not the entire amount of FM. There are fats which are essential to the body's health and maintenance) of FM. Setting this goal of 50lb weight loss will bring the total weight to 196lbs leaving 34lbs of FM. This 34lbs of FM brings this individual's body composition to 17% fat which is a healthy target for men. The importance of fat and its functions will be discussed in Chapter 5.

Equally, fat loss should not be the only goal, as it is important that muscle gain accompanies fat loss. Many obese individuals who only target fat in their weight loss journey usually end up having hanging and flabby skin causing them to feel unshapely. They failed to realize that muscle is a great contributor to the curves of the human body.

The perfect specific goal should be written similarly to the following:

It is my personal goal to lose 30lbs of fat and gain 5-10lbs of muscle. For the past few years I have been feeling heavier, less confident, and have trouble or just simply can't fit into my old clothes. I want to decrease my blood pressure and hopefully reduce the amount of daily medications. The areas where I hold the most fat are by arms, hips and stomach. The challenges I have to face and overcome in order to reach this goal are my cravings and busy schedule.

Write your goal here:

_____

_____

_____

_____

_____

_____

_____

_____

Measurable:

Creating a definable and tangible goal is critical to success. Measurements can be accounted for in two forms: a) setting a definition or criteria for what dictates whether you reach this goal or not b) setting checkpoints or short-term goals to measure progress towards accomplishing the goal.

A) When using objective goals, your criteria for success is often found within the goal itself. If your objective goal is to lose 30lbs, your measurement will be dictated by...losing 30lbs. The same is true if your goal is to increase your income by $1,000. When your pay stub includes an extra $1,000, obviously you have reached this goal.

Setting measurements for subjective goals can prove to be more difficult as some aspects within your goal may be quantifiable while others may not. If you choose a subjective goal such as being healthier, then you must first set the criteria by creating identifiable markers of this goal. Some identifiable contributors towards being healthier can include total weight, blood pressure reports, diabetes medication, energy level, how you feel when waking up in the morning, appearance and texture of skin, frequency of smiling and laughing, hair texture/breakage/new growth, exercise frequency, or even how long you can keep up with the kids. In general, you should be able to list what the contributing factors of your subjective goal.

I will measure my goal by (these should not be the goal itself but supporting criteria in rout to reaching your goal):

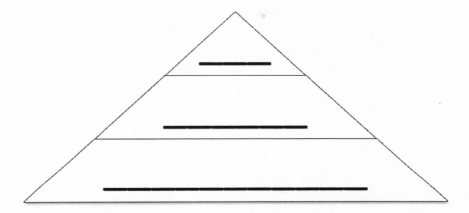

B) Setting checkpoints or benchmarks (at least 3) should be progressive steps on a staircase with the specific goal at its end. These benchmarks should be quantifiable or qualitative indicators leading to success.

Continuing with the above objective goal of losing 30lbs, measurements can reflect weight loss in increments of 10lbs or less. Your goal can also include different indicators such as pants/dress size, the buttons on your shirt fit differently, the ability to tuck in your shirt, fitting into your old jeans, you aren't out of breath when walking the stairs, using specific holes on your belt loop, smaller waist size or even shrinking your double chin etc.

These measurements can be written and accounted for in multiple ways, but I tend to favor the following:

Create a checklist (whether your goal is objective or subjective) with benchmarks or contributing factors towards your goal and check off each mark you reach and indicate the date and time.

Your checklist may resemble this (in no particular order):

- Lost 1 pants/dress size____
- My shirt buttons no longer stretched____

- I'm able to tuck in my shirt____
- I can now fit into my favorite gray jeans____
- I am using the 3rd belt hole and not the 2nd____
- My double chin no longer makes me uncomfortable____
- It is easier for me to put my dress shirts on in the morning__
- I have more energy____
- Lost 5lbs____
- Lost 10lbs____
- Lost 20lbs____
- Lost 30lbs____
- Lost 45lbs____

Create your own checklist:

Mark/circle the areas of your body where you would like to cut fat, gain muscle and/or slim down. Draw on the image and indicate exactly what changes you want to see and where.

___ Hands ___ Face ___ Lower Back

___ Wrists ___ Upper Chest ___ Upper Glutes

___ Forearm ___ Lower Chest ___ Lower Glutes

___ Biceps ___ Arm pit (anterior/posterior) ___ Hips/side of your butt

___ Triceps ___ Abdominal Area ___ Quadriceps

___ Shoulders ___ Upper Back ___ Hamstrings

___ Neck ___ Obliques/Love Handles ___ Calfs

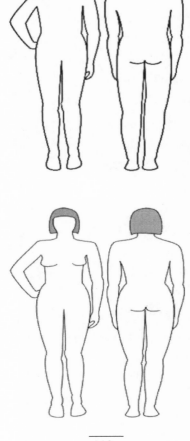

Attainable:

To make your goal attainable, ask yourself this question, "Is my goal realistic and how can I accomplish it?" Most people respond with a blanket "Yes", but are often unable to identify how they will achieve their goal. Think of it this way. If you are a 40-year-old janitor in a fortune 500 company with no degree, skills or relevant background, the attainability of becoming the Executive Director is extremely limited and not realistic.

In terms of setting health goals, it is important to make sure your goal is realistic. Once upon a time, I had a 33-year-old male client who was 5'7" and weighed 150lbs. When assessing his figure and muscle tone, he had little excess fat around his midsection, legs and arms. He was your typical skinny guy. His goal was to lose 30lbs bringing his weight to 120lbs. For most people, the health risks of this goal are obvious as he had very little fat to begin with. In order to reach his goal, he would be burning nearly 23lbs of muscle tissue and very little fat. But for this gentleman, he had a goal set in his mind, and a self-image branded in his imagination. He felt it was my duty to help him reach his goal regardless of his health. I explained and educated him as to why that goal was unhealthy and together we explored better avenues to reaching his true goal which was to change his appearance. As opposed to losing 30lbs, he gained 8lbs of muscle and became more satisfied with his appearance.

According the American Council on Exercise, many obesity experts have suggested adhering to a 10% weight loss over a 6 month period as this is a healthy and attainable way to reach and maintain weight loss. After achieving this 10% decrease in total weight loss, a re-evaluation of the initial goals (particularly weight loss goals) should be completed. Example, if you weigh 300lbs, with six months of exercise and healthy eating, you should have lost *at least* 30lbs of fat, which equates to 5lbs/month. Yes, this number may seem extremely low but the end goal is not only weight loss, but to create a new lifestyle of consistency. Recreate your habits and build a system for yourself and as you continue on this road to health, weight will continue to shed. Unfortunately, for many individuals engaging in "lose weight fast" programs, **2/3rds of weight is often regained within one year and almost all of it in five years** (Wadden et al. 1989).

According to the American College of Sports Medicine, it is healthy to lose 1-2lbs of fat per week. There are about 24 weeks in 6 months. The ability to remain consistent with healthy eating and exercise, can yield a weight loss of about 8lbs per month. Thus, your total weight loss can be 48lb in 6 months. As previously mentioned, due to the risks your body experiences with drastic weight fluctuations, two pounds per week is the maximum weight loss I suggest in a one week period.

After determining whether your goal is attainable in a healthy manner, setting action steps will lay the framework and answer the question, "How"?

You have set your goal, you have created benchmarks and checklists and now we need to determine how to get you started.

Starting my Step-By-Step plan

1. Become more active and health conscious on your own:

Before the gym membership and before the personal trainer, start becoming more active on your own which helps you to reset your mind. This mental refresh allows you to become more open to physical activity and also increases the chances you will maintain this new lifestyle.

Complete the form below entitled "Physical Activity Readiness Questionnaire" to determine how prepared your body is to exercise and any steps you may need to take engaging in an exercise plan.

PAR-Q & You

Physical Activity Readiness Questionnaire

The Physical Activity Readiness Questionnaire (PAR-Q) is designed to help you help yourself. Many health benefits are associated with regular exercise and completion of the PAR-Q is an essential first step to take if you are planning to increase the amount of physical activity in your life. For most people, physical activity should not pose any problem or hazard. The PAR-Q has be designed to identify the small number of adults for whom physical activity might be inappropriate or those who should seek medical advice concerning the type of activity most suitable for them.

NAME:_____ DATE:_____

HEIGHT: _____ in. WEIGHT: _____lbs. AGE: _____

PHYSICIANS NAME: _____ PHYSICIANS PHONE: _____

Common sense is your best guide in answering these questions. Please read them carefully and (X) the [] YES or [] NO opposite the question if it applies to you.

		YES	NO
1	Has your doctor ever said that you have a heart condition and that you should only perform physical activity recommended by a doctor?		
2	Do you feel pain in your chest when you perform physical activity?		
3	In the past month, have you had chest pain when you were not performing any physical activity?		
4	Do you lose your balance because of dizziness or do you ever lose consciousness?		
5	Do you have a bone or joint problem that could be made worse by a change in your physical activity?		

6	Is your doctor currently prescribing any medication for your blood pressure or for a heart condition?		
7	Do you know of any other reason why you should not engage in physical activity?		

If you have answered "Yes" to one or more of the above questions, consult your physician before engaging in physical activity. Tell your physician each "Yes" answer. After a medical evaluation, seek advice from your physician on what type of activity is suitable for your current condition.

After completing this form regardless of the results, I always suggest visiting your doctor. When visiting your physician make sure to retrieve blood work, weight and BMI scores along with your physical examination. Ask your physician for feedback on your goals as they may provide information that can be helpful in your weight loss journey.

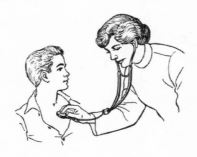

I am always interested in how my words have affected others. At this point, take a full body photo (front, side and back) and mark this date as your before photo: Date: _____. Since you have decided to enter into this journey with me lets track all of your progress. I will also ask you to take an after photo and submit it to me detailing your exercise journey and the results this book has allowed you to reach. I expect your results to be epic! For those with the most significant results and testimonies, I may just fly out to you and run you through a Coach Cailah training session! Imagine that. Let's get started!

2. The baby steps of increasing your activity

- Parking further away
- Taking short 5-10min walking breaks at work
- Taking the stairs (no matter how much extra time it takes)
- Playing with your kids
- Standing more often and sitting less, focusing on good posture
- Setting walking dates with friends and family
- Walking your dog
- Drinking more water
- Eating better foods
- Using less salt, using less fat in meal preparation
- Eating out less often
- In general being outside and in motion more often

Also, begin keeping a journal or food log of what you eat. This will help you track eating habits, which may vary due to daily changes in, emotions, and/or stress levels. Jot down what you consume, as you eat it. (See Chapter 5: Nutrition for food log).

Your goal in this stage is having the ability to walk for 10 minutes without rest at a consistent pace, and to have kept a food log for at least two weeks straight. After you become more comfortable with moving your body through multiple planes of motion at varying speeds and are more aware of the foods you eat, move to step three.

3. Find your exercise work place

Find a place where you do not mind getting a little dirty (literally and figuratively), and where excuses cannot find you. For some people, this is a gym membership because they don't like being outside. Others may find a park or a walking trail they enjoy. If you choose making your dedicated exercise location a park, track or other outdoor area, DO NOT let the rain, cold, or the sun deter you (safe weather conditions will be explained in chapter 6). If there is inclement weather, always have a backup plan, like the treadmill in your house that most of you don't use! If you choose the gym as your exercise work place, make certain you are comfortable with its entire environment, as to not let people hinder you from your goals.

Here are a few key items to look for when choosing a gym:

- Your determinants should include membership cost
- Member profiles (the type of people that gym caters towards)
- Cleanliness
- Staff visibility
- Interesting fitness classes (if desired)
- Daycare (if needed)

Once you have found the right fit, make friends with the staff. Good conversation and relationship building go a long way in keeping you accountable.

4. **Set your Workout Routine and create a nutrition accountability system**

As an overview, after you have become more physically active in step one, your body is now prepared for a more intensive mode of physical activity. Set your goal for a minimum of two days per week of exercise (whether at the gym or at the park), while performing a total of 30 minutes (mins) of physical activity in any form (playing with your kids, vigorous cleaning etc.) on all or most days of the week.

Example; hit the gym Mondays and Wednesdays while on Tuesday, Thursday and Saturday you walk, play "Dance Dance Revolution®", or

> **Design Your Body Challenge**
>
> Complete 150 minutes of Cardio within the next 4 days and list your time below.
> Day 1:_____
> Day 2:_____
> Day 3:_____
> Day 4:_____

simply enjoy an activity that keeps you moving. Details of how to create a workout routine that will help you reach your goals can be found in Chapters 6-8; Exercise.

Journaling your daily nutrition is important. After step one, you should have become more conscious of the types and qualities of the foods you consume. Now is the time to make changes. Set a plan to eat right six days a week and have a "light" cheat day on day seven. Food should not be the only reward in your plan but if that reward consists of diner and a movie, well, it's okay to have a little extra butter on your popcorn!

Chapter 5 on Nutrition will help you outline specific calorie goals for your body type and goals. This is what you will use to track your nutrition.

Relevant:

Your goal should be extremely important and personal to you. The relevancy of your goal will help drive you towards success. If one of your benchmark goals is to look great in a new suit that's two sizes smaller than your current size, the specifics and measurability of you accomplishing this goal need to support your goal in its entirety. Yes buying the new slacks or a dress helps, but every detail needs to strongly support making this goal become a reality.

Your goal should reflect the outcomes that you want to see. Relevant goals typically answer these questions:

- Is it worthwhile?
- Is this the right time?
- Are you able to put forth the necessary effort?
- Do you have the right support?

Timely:

This category tends to be particularly tricky with attempting weight loss. Question: Is it possible to drop 20lbs in 1 month? Answer: Yes it is. Fact: This weight loss can happen with certain body types, but usually it is extremely unhealthy. Many individuals who experience extreme weight loss in a short period of time gain back the weight they lost and often times much more. Another Fact: It is extremely difficult to lose 20lbs in 30days. That boils down to 2/3rds of a pound every day equating to a total calorie burn of 2333 calories per day! This is extremely unsafe and dangerous for most people and only occurs in controlled environments.

A safe rule-of-thumb is 5-8lbs of weight loss per month. If your goal is to lose 30lbs, than your goal should to be set for six months or more. You must understand that this is a journey down the yellow brick road. At times, you will see munchkins, fairies, phony magicians and wicked witches, but as long as you stay the course, we'll get to Kansas together.

Long-Term goal:

My long-term weight loss goal is _____ lbs.
I will reach this goal in _____ months weeks years (circle)

Short-term goals/benchmarks:

I will reach my benchmark 1 goal by _____ (write a date)
I will reach my benchmark 2 goal by _____ (write a date)
I will reach my benchmark 4 goal by _____ (write a date)

Design Your Body Fitness Challenge: Make A Plan

One of the biggest issues with exercise that people have is that it doesn't fit within their schedule. For this week's Design Your Body Fitness Challenge, I challenge you to sit down and write out your own exercise schedule.

Your schedule runs your life, so once you take ownership of it, you will then have full control. Write down a day by day schedule and plot your exercise. The goal is to exercise a BARE MINIMUM of 4 days/week.

Post a pic of your exercise schedule on my page and keep me updated on your completion. Without accountability, tasks often don't get accomplished.

I CHALLENGE YOU to post your exercise schedule on my page and I WILL help you stay accountable to it!

Keep up with me and watch me keep up with you!

Stay tuned for my upcoming book on Weight Loss.

Design Your Body

CHAPTER 3

Finding Your Starting Line

Now that you have set your goals and you have clear indicators as how to maintain success, it's time to walk to the tack and find exactly your starting line. This chapter will aid you in assessing your current health/ fitness status and show you a direct path for the steps you need to take in starting your exercise program.

Obesity is an epidemic sweeping the world while heavily concentrated in the United States. This disease is a serious threat to your health and exposes you to medical risks such as diabetes, dyslipidemia/ hypercholesterolemia, gallbladder disease, arthritis, hypertension and various forms of cancer. The economic, medical and psychological costs of maintaining health in our country have drastically increased. A recent study conducted by the National Health and Nutrition Examination Survey found that 68.3% of adults age 20 and older are overweight or obese. The rates of obese in individuals, age 40-59 have risen to 77.8% in males while 66.3% in females. Concerning race and ethnicity in adults 20 years and older, non-Hispanic whites have the lowest statistics of obesity at 67.5% while non-Hispanic blacks rank 73.7% and Mexican Americans at 77.5% (ACE - American Council on Exercise, 2011, p. 201). In every population mentioned above the health risks are over 60%!

Choosing an appropriate starting line is a significant step in the right direction toward accomplishing the goals you created above. It is imperative to know as much as possible about your medical/physical state in preparation for creating an exercise plan (detailed in chapters 6-8) that will not only effectively combat your current condition in a healthy and safe manner, but with help you begin the road to 'Designing Your Body'.

But What If I Fail!?

The thought of failure is one of the scariest things about beginning a new journey. Thoughts may flood your mind with what ifs, embarrassments, setbacks, relapses, low confidence and dozens of self-defeating statements. The fact is that your road to health is not a direct path. Expect detours, pit stops, and wrong turns from friends, family and sometimes even yourself. Yes, it's true, there will be times when you defeat yourself, but the goal is not to remain defeated. When you mess up, accept your actions, note how and what led you to that point, then get up, shake yourself off and, as my mother would say, "Keep on Stepping!"

What does it look like? Self-defeat can resemble a cheat snack turning into a cheat meal, then a cheat day; or you may not exercise for an entire week! However, as long as you do not stay defeated, you will continue to progress. It is better to inch forward than to jump in place. Set progress as your goal and never be stagnant, always move forward.

In order to minimize failure, because it will happen, make a list of things that will tempt you to relapse into old habits. These things can be cheesecake, Swedish Fish, an old girlfriend, cookouts, vacations, office parties, going to a buffet etc.

My List of Temptations:

_____	_____	_____
_____	_____	_____
_____	_____	_____
_____	_____	_____
_____	_____	_____
_____		

"Our greatest glory is not in never failing, but
in rising up every time we fail."
-Ralph Waldo Emerson

Determining Your Risk Factors

As we age, eat, decrease activity and become consistently more sedentary in our desk jobs and rudimentary routines. We have either contracted various cardiovascular diseases due to the negative habits we have created, or we have put ourselves at risk for developing these diseases. Though you are excited about losing weight, we must determine where you currently rank on a physiological/medical level to determine what types of exercise are best for you before we begin.

Developing atherosclerotic or other cardiovascular diseases (CVD) are a serious matter. Most of these diseases can be reversed by proper nutritional and exercise lifestyle changes (notice the word "diet" is not mentioned). All individuals, healthy or not, are placed in one of three risk categories for developing a CVD; 1) low, 2) moderate, or 3) high risk. The process by which individuals are assigned to one of these risk categories is based on;

a). The presence or absence of a known CVD, pulmonary and or/ metabolic disease
b). The presence or absence of signs or symptoms suggestive of CVD, pulmonary and/or metabolic disease and/or
c). The presence or absence of CVD risk factors (ACSM, 2010, p. 22)

Low Risk: Individuals classified in this category either do not have any signs or symptoms of or have not been diagnosed with a CVD, pulmonary and/or metabolic disease as well has having one or less risk factor for CVD. Individuals in this category have a low risk for experiencing a cardiovascular event and an exercise program can be pursued safely without the need of clearance or a medical examination from your physician (ACSM, 2010, p. 22).

Moderate Risk: Individuals listed as Moderate Risk do not have any signs/symptoms of, nor have they been diagnosed with CVD, pulmonary, and/or metabolic diseases but they have two or more positive risk factors. The risk of experiencing a cardiovascular event in this population has increased due to the multiple positive risk factors associated with these individuals. Though the risk is higher in this category, in most cases, these individuals may safely participate in low to moderate intensity exercise without the need of clearance or a medical examination from your physician. It is still advised to have a medical examination and an exercise test before participating in high intensity exercises (greater than 60% of maximal exertion) (ACSM, 2010, p. 23).

High Risk: Being classified as high risk is determined by having one or more sign/symptom of or being diagnosed with a current CVD, pulmonary, and/or metabolic diseases. The risk of a cardiovascular event for these individuals is increased to the point where a medical examination and exercise test should occur before the onset of exercise (ACSM, 2010, p. 23). After being cleared for exercise, I recommend physicians supervision or the oversight of a certified personal trainer if you identify as high risk.

The below table indicates positive risk factors for CVD set forth by the American College of Sports Medicine (ACSM, 2010, p. 28). Review each category and determine if you fall within the qualifying marks of the defining criteria. For example, if you are a 48-year-old man who is a current smoker, you have a positive risk factor for both Age and Smoking based upon the criteria set below, ranking you in the moderate risk category as the number of positive risk factors is summed.

Atherosclerotic Cardiovascular Disease
(CVD) Risk Factor Thresholds

Positive Risk Factors	Defining Criteria
Age	Men $\geq$ 45yr; Women $\geq$ 55yr
Family History	Having any close relative who has suffered a myocardial infarction, coronary revascularization, or sudden death before 55yr of age in father or other male first-degree relative, or before 65yr of age in mother or other female first-degree relative
Cigarette Smoking	Current cigarette smoker or those who quit within the previous 6 months or exposure to environmental tobacco smoke
Sedentary Lifestyle	Not participating in at least 30mins of moderate intensity (40-60% of max effort) physical activity on at least three days per week for at least 3 months
Obesity	Body mass index $\geq$ 30 or waist girth > 102cm (40in) for men and > 88cm (35in) for women
Hypertension/High Blood Pressure	Systolic blood pressure $\geq$140mmGh and/or diastolic blood pressure $\geq$ 90mmHg confirmed by measurements on at least two separate occasions
Dyslipidemia	Low-density lipoprotein (LDL-C) cholesterol $\geq$130mg.dL-1 (3.37mmol.L-1) or high-density lipoprotein (HDL-C) cholesterol < 40mg.dL-1 (1.04mmol.L-1) or on lipid-lowering medication. If total serum cholesterol is all that is available, use $\geq$ 200mg.dL-1 (5.18mmol.L-1)
Prediabetes	Impaired fasting glucose (IFG) = fasting plasma glucose $\geq$100mg.dL-1 (5.5mmol.L-1) but <126mg.dL-1 (6.93mmol.L-1) or impaired glucose tolerance (IGT) = 2-hour values in oral glucose tolerance test (OGTT) $\geq$140mg.dL-1 (7.70mmol.L-1) but <200mg.dL-1 (11.0mmol.L-1) confirmed by measurements on at least two separate occasions
Negative Risk Factor	Defining Criteria
High-serum HDL cholesterol	$\geq$60mg.dL -1 (1.55mmol.L-1)

(ACSM, 2010, p. 28)

Possessing three or more CVD risk factors can indicate the diagnosis of Metabolic Syndrome. The International Diabetes Federation (IDF) has proposed another definition for metabolic syndrome which can be categorized as the presence of abdominal adiposity and two additional CVD risk factors. There are three suggested treatment methods for Metabolic Syndrome according to the National Centers for Environmental Prediction:

1. Weight control
2. Physical activity
3. Treatment of represented CVD risk factors which may include physician recommended medication.

Major Signs or Symptoms Suggestive of Cardiovascular, Pulmonary or Metabolic Disease

Sign or Symptom	Definition/Significance
Pain, discomfort in the chest, neck, jaw, arms or other areas resulting in ischemia	This is one of the cardinal manifestations of cardiac disease, specifically coronary artery disease. Is provoked by exercise or exertion, excitement, cold or other forms of stress.
Shortness of breath at rest or with mild exertion	Dyspnea is defined as abnormally uncomfortable awareness of breathing. Abnormal exertional dyspnea suggests the presence of cardiopulmonary disorders, specifically, left ventricular dysfunction or COPD.
Dizziness or Syncope	Syncope is defined as a loss of consciousness and is most commonly caused by a reduction in blood flow to the brain. Dizziness and syncope during exercise may result from cardiac
Orthopnea or Paroxysmal Nocturnal Dyspnea	Orthopnea refers to dyspnea occurring at rest in a reclined position and is relieved by sitting upright or standing. Paroxysmal nocturnal dyspnea refers to dyspnea occurring 2-5hrs after the onset of sleep. Both are symptoms of left ventricular dysfunction.
Ankle Edema	Bilateral ankle edema is most evident at night and is characteristic of heart failure or bilateral chronic pooling and insufficient blood return within the veins. Unilateral edema of a
Palpitations or Tachycardia	Palpitations are defined as an unpleasant awareness of the strong and rapid beating of the heart. Tachycardia is an extremely rapid beating of the heart ≥ 100bpm

Intermittent Claudication	Refers to the pain that occurs in a muscle due to an inadequate blood supply that is further stressed by exercise. This is usually a result of atherosclerosis. This pain does not occur with standing or sitting and is reproducible day-to-day. Pain is severe when walking up stairs or uphill. Coronary artery disease is usually present within individuals presenting with Intermittent Claudication.
Known heart murmur	Some heart murmurs may be innocent, while others may indicate valvular or other CVD
Usual fatigue or shortness of breath with usual activities	Though certain instances of this issue may be benign, they also may signal the onset of, or change in the status of cardiovascular, pulmonary or metabolic disease.

(ACSM, 2010, pp. 26-27)

Based on the above charts I am categorized as (circle one):

    a.   Low Risk and I can begin exercise immediately.

          a.   I've not been diagnosed with a CVD, nor do I have any signs or symptoms of a CVD and I have < 2 risk factors.

    b.   Moderate Risk and I can engage in low to moderate intensity exercise (40-60% of maximal effort).

          a.   I've not been diagnosed with a CVD, nor do I have any signs or symptoms of a CVD but I have ≥ 2 risk factors.

    c.   High Risk and I should consult a physician to receive a medical examination and clearance before I begin my physical activity.

          a.   I have ≥ 1 sign or symptom of a CVD, and/or I have been diagnosed with a CVD, pulmonary and/or metabolic disease. This category is not dependent upon risk factors as the signs or symptoms are indicators of disease.

After discovering your risk stratification you are better equip to choose the best path and tempo for beginning and creating an exercise program that best suits you and allow you to maximize your training efforts.

What do you do if you have two or more CVD risk factors after seeing your physician?

1. Reduce the amount of calories you intake
2. Increase physical activity to 30minutes/day 5-7days/week
3. Improve the quality of foods you eat.

Design Your Body Fitness Challenge: Free Your Mind!

This week's challenge is to participate in 60 minutes of an activity that's outside of your norm. Yoga and other Mind/Body style exercises aren't my favorite (I'm more of a weight room chick) but I cannot deny the extremely positive health benefits they have (decreased stress levels, increased breath control, flexibility, balance and strength). Get out this week and participate in different types of exercises that stray away from your typical routine.

   I Challenge You! Post your pictures of your new/different exercise on my Facebook wall.

The Big Deal with Blood Pressure

Most of us know the goal blood pressure (BP) reading is 120/80 and that our readings shouldn't rise above this figure. But many cannot define BP nor how it is manipulated. Many are also not aware that it can be regulated without medication. Systolic pressure (the top number) is literally the amount of pressure or resistance within the arteries that your heart has to overcome in order to pump its next pool of blood to the entire body. Diastolic pressure is the amount of pressure or resistance in the veins as blood returns to the heart.

The higher the systolic and diastolic figures (often due to decreases arteriole elasticity and increased plaque buildup), the more at risk you are for experiencing a cardiovascular event (any occurrence that causes damage to the heart muscle) independent of other CVD risk factors. For individuals age 40-70, every 20mmHg (millimeters of mercury) in systolic BP or 10mmHg in diastolic BP doubles the risk of cardiovascular disease (ACSM, 2010, p. 47).

Blood Pressure Classification for Adults Age 18 and Older

Category	Systolic (mmHg)	Diastolic (mmHg)	Begin Exercise
Normal	<120	<80	Yes
Prehypertension	120-139	80-89	Yes, between 40-60% of maximal intensity. Consult a physician. Lifestyle modification needed.
Stage 1 hypertension	140-159	90-99	Yes, only low intensity exercises should be performed on your own while moderate-high intensity programs should only be performed under professional supervision (trainer, physician etc.). Lifestyle modification needed.
Stage 2 hypertension	≥160	≥100	Consult your physician before you begin any activity. Lifestyle modification required.

Please note that the use of beta blockers will effect BP readings. Blood pressure readings should be read on two separate occasions, on the same arm after two minutes of sitting still with feet flat on the floor for, and with your arms not crossed accurate measurements.

The Danger of Obesity

Being "big boned" is no longer an excuse for accumulated fat. Identifying yourself as "full figured" or "thick" does not make it OK to be overweight. Outside of the physical personal discomfort many experience with being overweight, it is extremely dangerous, and can cause life-threatening complications that could otherwise be prevented.

Obesity is directly linked to several chronic diseases including CVD, type II diabetes mellitus, various forms of cancer, and an abundance of muscular and skeletal problems. Being over fat exposes you, regardless of age, to many preventable diseases. Wake up and do something about your health, happiness and future!

"An ounce of prevention is worth a pound of cure."
— Benjamin Franklin

John was a former client of mine who was obese. His main goal in working with me wasn't for aesthetics, but it was because he understood that eventually his habits would lead to his death. He feared that he would not see his son or daughter (3 and 5 at the time) grow into adulthood. John was as strong as an ox, very tall but had a tire belly. My goal with John was not to get him stronger, but to reduce the fat around his abdominal section, which is identified as android obesity (android obesity = apple shaped while gynoid obesity = pear shaped as the fat is stored in the hips, buttocks thighs and lower stomach. Those who suffer from android obesity are at a higher risk for disease). After we completed the necessary paperwork, cardio and interval training became John's best friend. We walked with intermittent speed walks, climbed stairs with plenty of breaks, hit the Stairmaster, elliptical and treadmill all while incorporating endurance style resistance training (higher repetitions and lower weights). John lost inches off his midsection, increased the strength in his legs and arms, was able to run consistently for almost 3 miles at a good pace and is still living a happy and healthy life watching his family grow.

It is important to note where your fat storage sites are (saying, "EVERYWHERE!" doesn't count). Some may carry fat in their arms, hips, stomach or thighs, which all have specific health status indicators. If the majority of your stored fat is located in the abdominal area (android obesity, apple-shape) you are at a higher risk of developing:

a. Coronary heart disease
b. High BP
c. High cholesterol
d. Type II diabetes
e. Stroke

This differs for persons who gain a majority of their weight in their thighs and buttocks (gynoid obesity, pear-shape).

This fact indicates that it is extremely important to track your waist and hip circumferences to determine your potential for developing an obesity related disease (outside of previously stated CVD risk factors that indicate what is already present). The measurement of your waist and hips can help indicate your potential/risk level for developing an obesity related disease and is simply called Waist to Hip Ratio. This calculation is performed by dividing waist circumference by hip circumference (waist/hip = wait to hip ratio) and you will often see me notate this waist W: H.

When measuring your waist, women, take a horizontal measurement at the narrowest part of the torso above the umbilicus (belly button) and below the xiphoid process. Men, take your measurement at the level of the umbilicus. The hip measurement should be done horizontally at the maximal circumference of the gluteus maximus. Divide your waist circumferences in (inches) by hip circumferences (inches) and find your ranking below.

As we continue to identify your starting place, we need to clearly indicate your weight, and circumferences. You will see this Weight Check throughout the book as a means to keep yourself progressing as you read this book.

Weight Check:

My current weight is: _____lbs x 2.2lbs/kg is: _____ kg, Today's date: _____

My waist circumference is: _____inches, Today's date: _____

My hip circumference is: _____inches, Today's date: _____

Waist-to-Hip Ratio

Gender	Excellent	Good	Average
Male	<0.85	0.85-0.89	0.90-0.94
Female	<0.75	0.75-0.79	0.80-0.85

Your weight fluctuates in response to the simple ratio of energy balance. As you will see in a later section (The All Mighty Calorie) calories are energy and in order to maintain weight, calories that enter your body should = calories burned by the body. If you intake more calories than you burn than you are in a positive caloric balance and those calories will be stored as fat and you will gain weight. If you burn more calories than you intake, you will be in a negative caloric balance and you will lose weight. For obese individuals, in order to effectively manage your body weight, you must burn more calories (via exercise and physical activity) than what is added. A weight loss of 5-10% provides significant health benefits (such as reducing risk factors for CVD, potentially eradicating diabetes and removing hypertension just to name a few) and is the healthy figure you should target. The pace to set for reaching this goal is losing 1-2lbs/week. Weight loss programs that include a decrease in calorie intake along with an increase in calorie expenditure typically result in an *initial* 9-10% reduction in body weight. Write your target weight loss below.

5% of my current weight is: _____
10% of my current weight is: _____

Whether you are obese, overweight or over fat, this categorization is not based on the total number represented on the scale, but on the major components of your body (fat & fat free weight) that make up your total weight. If you weigh 244lbs, there is a certain percentage of you that is pure fat and another percentage that represents fat free mass (muscle, organ tissue, water & bone). We call this comparison Body Fat Percentage (BF %). It is fairly easy to find your BF%, most gyms have a handheld device with silver handles that you hold for a few seconds and it shows a percentage of you that is all fat (some devices are also weight scales and ask you to stand on them). Though not completely accurate, this is a good start. Again, if you weigh 244lbs, and your BF % reads 37%, this means that you have 90lbs of pure fat (244lbs X .37 = 90.28), and this is the weight that you should focus on losing. After you have calculated your total fat, it is important to note that there are optimal levels of fat that should remain in your body, and your goal should not be to become fat free.

Continuing in this example and referring back to our goals, if you have 90lbs of fat, and you currently weigh 244lbs, it is not healthy to set your goal weight at 160lbs, and possibly not even 170lbs. There is a certain amount of fat (dependent upon each individual) that is generally healthy for you to maintain. Also remember, women will, and are supposed to have more fat than men.

Percent Body Fat Norms for Men and Women

Category	Women	Men
Essential Fat	8-13%	2-5%
Athletes	14-20%	6-13%
Fitness	21-24%	24-27%
Acceptable/Normal	25-31%	18-24%
Obese	≥32%	≥25%

(ACE - American Council on Exercise, 2011, p. 236)

After engaging in a weight loss routine, managing the weight lost will be difficult, but you must stay the course and Don't Quit!

Approximately 33-50% of individuals who lost weight and discontinued exercise gained back the weight they lost, and many even gained more. Weight loss should become your goal until you reach that 5-10% figure, and then, staying fit and active should become your lifestyle. This journey has no end, there is only a beginning.

Body Mass Index

Body Mass Index (BMI) is a figure used for assistance in determining overall health status and serves as an estimate of body composition. The higher your BMI, the more at risk you are for developing obesity related diseases such as arthritis, heart disease, Type II Diabetes, gallstones, hypertension (high BP), and stroke.

Though BMI is not the sole indicator of health status, it is a quick and simple way to generalize health status. Because BMI is a ratio of height and weight, there are some individuals who fall within undesirable BMI ranges but who are completely healthy. As an example, most bodybuilders are overweight when categorized in terms of BMI due to their total weight in relation to their height.

Body Mass Index is a figure calculated by dividing body weight (in kilograms kg) into height^2 (in meters m^2).

$$BMI = \frac{Weight(kg)}{(Height^2\ (m)}$$

Take Sarah who is 5'11" and 180lbs.

- Step 1, convert weight in pounds to kilograms (kg) by dividing her weight by 2.2 (187lbs/2.2 = 85kg).
- Step 2, convert height from total inches into centimeters by multiplying height in inches by 2.54cm then dividing by 100cm/m (5'11" → 71in x 2.54cm = 180.34cm/100(cm/m) = 1.8034m).
- Step 3, divide weight into height^2 (85kg/1.8034m^2) =BMI

BMI Reference Chart

Weight Range	BMI
Underweight	<18.5
Normal Weight	18.5-24.9
Overweight	25.0-29.9
Grade I Obesity	35.0-34.9
Grade II Obesity	35.0-39.9
Morbid Obesity	≥40

What is your BMI _____ date: _____
goal BMI: _____

To save you the trouble of calculating your own BMI, use the chart below

BODY MASS INDEX														
	Normal						Overweight					Obese		
BMI	19	20	21	22	23	24	25	26	27	28	29	30	35	40
Height (inches)	Weight (pounds)													
58	91	95	100	105	110	115	119	124	129	134	138	143	167	191
59	94	99	104	109	114	119	124	128	133	138	143	148	173	198
60	97	102	107	112	118	123	128	133	138	143	148	153	179	204
61	100	106	111	116	121	127	132	137	143	148	153	158	185	211
62	104	109	115	120	125	131	136	142	147	153	158	164	191	218
63	107	113	118	124	130	135	141	146	152	158	163	169	197	225
64	110	116	122	128	134	140	145	151	157	163	169	174	203	233
65	114	120	126	132	138	144	150	156	162	168	174	180	210	240
66	117	124	130	136	142	148	155	161	167	173	179	185	216	247
67	121	127	134	140	147	153	159	166	172	178	185	191	223	255
68	125	131	138	144	151	158	164	171	177	184	190	197	230	263
69	128	135	142	149	155	162	169	176	182	189	196	203	237	270
70	132	139	146	153	160	167	174	181	188	195	202	209	243	278
71	136	143	150	157	165	172	179	186	193	200	207	215	250	286
72	140	147	155	162	169	177	184	191	199	206	213	221	258	294
73	144	151	159	166	174	182	189	197	204	212	219	227	265	303
74	148	155	163	171	179	187	194	202	210	218	225	233	272	311
75	152	160	168	176	184	192	200	208	216	224	232	240	279	319
76	156	164	172	180	189	197	205	213	221	230	238	246	287	328

Note: Find your client's height in the far left column and move across the row to the weight that is closest to the client's weight. His or her body mass index will be at the top of that column.

(Exercise, 2013)

PART II

Design Your Body

CHAPTER 4

The Trinity of Health and Wellness

Being healthy requires a lasting marriage between multiple facets of health, but unfortunately many people often focus only on one or two aspects. When you consider being healthy, what does it consist of? Fewer doctor visits, higher energy levels, ridding yourself of metabolic diseases (hypertension, diabetes, obesity and each of their symptoms), no smoking, wiser alcohol intake, better sleep habits, whiter eyes, and healthier skin, nails and hair? Many of you will agree with these statements, each of which can be addressed with understanding of and operating within The Trinity of Health and Wellness.

With any trinity, there are three separate parts which if accomplished separately will benefit you to a certain level, but when accomplished as a unit in its entirety, you are able to operate and achieve success that was previously unavailable to you. Achieving working levels in the Trinity of Health and Wellness will help you achieve your goal of being a healthier and happier individual. Through all of my studies I have found these three things to be the collective key to attaining good health: Nutrition, Cardiovascular Endurance and Resistance Training. With these three, your goal can be achieved.

Notice I substituted the word 'diet' for nutrition as a 'diet' is a temporary change in eating habits. A diet is nothing more than a nutritional fad and something intending to be temporary! When I train for competitions, photo shoots or summer vacation, I put myself on a diet because the changes I am making are only temporary and for short term gain. You can stick to a diet if you want your weight loss to be temporary.

Also notice I have broken down the term 'exercise' as many people do not understand the physiological importance of versatility. If you work in a mail room where you lift boxes and push carts, the first day on the job is going to be physically demanding if you are not used to this activity. But after a few days of repetition, the task gets easier, not due to the load being lightened, but due to you becoming stronger. After working in the mail room for a few weeks, the stress on your body has diminished as your body has adapted to a new demand. If there is no change in demand, your body will remain the same.

On the same note, if you are an avid walker and the only exercise you participate in is walking, you are restricting your potential for weight loss! Yes cardio alone is still a great means of burning calories, but eventually, your body will adapt to the physiological stress of walking and it will not be *as* beneficial as when you first began. Again, when you grow to the point where your body has adapted to the stress of walking and if a new challenge isn't introduced, you, your progress and weight loss will plateau. You must add good nutrition and a solid resistance training program that will increase the calories you burn due to forcing the body to adapt to a new stressor. More calories burned = more fat lost.

Men, if all you do is hit upper body in the gym, not only will you look like Johnny Bravo, but

Design Your Body Challenge

Every morning immediately after you wake, and every night before bed, you must do 50 Squats or 50 push-ups for the next 7 days. Check off the days below.

Day 1: _____
Day 2: _____
Day 3: _____
Day 4: _____
Day 5: _____
Day 6: _____
Day 7: _____

you begin weakening your cardiovascular system due to inactivity. Yes, weightlifting burns calories, but the only way to maximize calorie burn is by adding in a nutritional lifestyle change and good solid cardio.

Most people focus on excelling at one aspect of The Trinity and wonder why they aren't reaching their goals of weight loss. The principle I am referring to is entitled **Specific Adaptations for Imposed Demand**. Plainly stated, your body will adapt to the stress and only the specific stress (exercise is a stress – think of the result of exercise as cause and effect, or even supply and demand as you are supplying your body with a stressor and demanding for it to change) that is applied to it. You may wish for a different outcome, but if you push the 7th floor on an elevator, it will only go to the 7th floor. Weight loss does not come from cardio, resistance training or good nutrition alone, you must tie all three aspects of health together in order to successfully reach your expected weight loss.

The Trinity Figures Scale

The Trinity Figures Scale is a ranking tool I created to help you quantify your current status in the areas of Nutrition, Cardiovascular Exercise and Resistance Training. How do you rate in The Trinity? Complete the below Trinity Figures Scale and rate yourself based upon the level you most consistently identify within Nutrition, Cardiovascular Endurance and Resistance Training. Use this rating system periodically to assess your progress in each area. This will assist you in keeping all areas balanced and consistently progressing.

Poor: 1-4 Average: 5-7 Good: 8-9 Excellent: 10

Nutrition:

1. I barely eat. I'm too busy or just not hungry.
2. My nutrition is trash. I still run for the ice-cream truck with a fast food burger in my hand.

3. I skip meals but overload at dinner.

4. I am a carnivore!

5. I eat when I can and try to make healthy choices. My healthy choices look like whatever is on the menu of the next fast food restaurant.

6. I eat a salad every now-and-again, but I have major weaknesses with carbs and sweets.

7. I get about two full meals per day. During my two meals I make sure I fill up!

8. I eat 3 square meals a day and don't skip meals but my portion control isn't the greatest. Some meals are frozen dinners but I'm improving. Plenty of water.

9. I eat 3 square meals and snack on whatever I can in-between. Plenty of water.

10. I eat 5-6 times a day with dairy, veggies, fruits, nuts, grains and healthy proteins in each meal. I time my meals to be 3-4 hours in-between to stay on schedule. Plenty of water.

Cardiovascular Endurance:

1. Huh? What is cardio? The only time I get my heart rate up is during rush hour traffic.

2. I park in the closest spot at work, do very little physical activity and never take the stairs.

3. I try and stand up or walk around my office when I get the chance.

4. I purposefully park far away to get more walking in but nothing else.

5. Every now and again I am pretty active with physical activity or sports but I can easily fall off my regimen.

6. I just started a new routine and I try to take part cardio 1-2 times per week for at least 30mins and try to stick to this regimen, I may fall off track but I try my best to get back on quickly.

7. I participate in cardio > 2 times per week for at least 30mins. I'm building the consistency of my exercise schedule.

8. I have a set regimen of cardio for at least 30mins > 3 days per week.

9. I engage in multiple types of cardio, walking, running, biking, swimming, hiking etc. more than 5 times per week.

10. I compete in and train for events, sports games, competitions (5k, basketball team, 10k etc.) or I'm on a team who practices 5+ days/week.

Resistance Training:

1. All I lift is my fork to my mouth.

2. I do minor things such as weekly cleaning, cooking, or caretaking.

3. I only do body weight exercises with not a lot of intensity such as Yoga but only when I get a chance.

4. I'm working on my schedule but when I go to the gym, I don't know what to do so I workout on machines, or I watch YouTube® exercise videos at home.

5. I'm becoming more consistent with my schedule, looking up exercises and I resistance train > 1 time per week. I may not know everything about resistance training but I'm faithful!

6. I spot train. I typically exercise certain muscle groups like upper body only or abs only. I don't focus on my legs and I'm not a fan of whole body activities.

7. While on my schedule I lift heavy weight low reps.

8. While on my schedule I lift light weight and lots of reps. I like the group classes at my gym or the group exercise sessions with friends.

9. I train for performance to increase muscle size, power and functional movement.

10. Olympic lifting is like my first-born child. I don't have to be a body builder but I want to be strong.

Your Ratings:

Nutrition: _____   Cardiovascular Endurance_____   Resistance Training_____

      Date: _____   Current Weight: _____

Nutrition: _____   Cardiovascular Endurance_____   Resistance Training_____

      Date: _____   Current Weight: _____

Nutrition: _____   Cardiovascular Endurance_____   Resistance Training_____

      Date: _____   Current Weight: _____

Nutrition: _____   Cardiovascular Endurance_____   Resistance Training_____

      Date: _____   Current Weight: _____

Every two months you should return to the Trinity Figures Scale and reassess your progress. This will allow you to adjust your training and nutrition program based upon your results. In other words, you should be changing or diversifying (i.e. increasing intensity, duration, and variation) your workout routine every 6-8 weeks. The adjustment will decrease the staleness of your workouts and help combat plateauing. Your goal is to move from your current rating and become well rounded in each area of the Trinity of Health, Wellness and Fitness. Reach for rankings of 8 or higher which categorizes you as "Good" mark for each area.

Let's Consider Sam:

Sam is a 43 year old Yoga instructor who teaches 3-4 classes each week for about 1hr each session for his exercise. He also has excellent nutrition as he strictly believes in eating six small meals, loading up on fruits/veggies, light on the carbs, good sources of protein such as chicken and seafood and plenty of water. The issue, is that Sam recently lost weight and has extra skin around his arms, chest and midsection, but still isn't where he wants to be physically. Sam is succeeding with Nutrition management, lacking in Resistance Training and his Cardio is non-existent. Though Yoga is an extremely beneficial style of exercise, it should not be his only form of exercise.

Resistance training is the most important type of activity Sam should engage in. He has lost a significant amount of weight but has only lost fat and not built the extra muscle necessary to create a shapely and defined body. Those who lose weight often see sagging skin as a result of the skin being stretched around the extra mass. Upon weight loss, the skin remains stretched and begins to sag due to gravity. The best way to combat this issue is resistance training to build muscle tone which will add shape and definition to the body.

Yes, Yoga is technically a form of resistance training as you fight gravity to maintain various body weight poses. The downfall with those who only participate in Yoga is that the body is no longer forced to adapt as it is not challenged by activity. As he ages, without proper resistance training Sam's body will remain nimble due to Yoga but he will still be as likely to injure himself with bone breaks/fractures should he fall. Yoga will improve your balance, proprioception, flexibility, blood flow, breathing and posture (along with many other benefits). Unfortunately, it will not improve bone mineral density (BMD is the density of your bones: the more dense they are, the harder it is to injure or break), nor speed, power or agility. Without speed, power or agility you cannot catch yourself in a fall, or quickly support yourself in times of need…Selah.

Sam also needs to add a Cardiovascular Training program as cardio can serve as an extreme calorie-burning tool to help him shed his remaining pounds. If he adds running or any other weight-baring activity into his regime, it will also help increase his bone mineral density as the body will be forced to adapt to the positive stressors that have been added a.k.a. running.

Sam's Trinity Figures Scale rankings: Currently Sam's Nutrition = 9/10, Resistance Training =5/10 and Cardiovascular Endurance =0/10.

If Sam adds resistance training (either before or after he teaches Yoga) to his regimen to improve his muscle tone, he will increase his definition and reduce his skin sagging. He also needs to add a weight-baring cardio routine to further all enhancements seen in resistance training and Yoga (particular health benefits of cardio will be discussed in the Cardiovascular Endurance chapter), along with assisting with extra calorie burn to reach his fitness goal.

There will be certain areas where you excel and others where you fall short. Use your Trinity Figures Scale to determine which areas need to improve and by what margin. In the following chapters, I provide specific information as how to move from one figure to the next. This will be key in helping you create your own plan.

CHAPTER 5

Nutrition

I am not a registered dietitian. I do recognize that some individuals may have specific health requirements that fall outside the following scientifically proven information and recommendations. I strongly recommend you consult a dietitian if you feel these suggestions will not benefit you.

Eating healthy is not like peering into a mirror that shows another dimension where dogs walk people, raccoons are pets, slugs are bosses and humans are cone headed aliens who speak like Lieutenant Commander Data from Star Trek™. Eating healthy is actually a fairly easy thing to do. Most of us blame our lack of healthy eating on our schedules as we feel we are too busy to cook, too busy to prepare lunches, or too busy to sit down and eat dinner as a family. That's rubbish! You should make your schedule work for you, rather than letting your schedule run you. In the end, you are the one who will have to pay for your medical expenses due to a lifetime of unhealthy living. Taking the extra time on your health will pave the way for your future, as well as the future of your family (especially if you have kids who are watching your every move and adopting your eating habits). Peering into the mirror should not be amplified by the fear of not knowing what's healthy, what to eat, when to eat it, what's right, wrong, good bad, etc. Peering into the mirror should reflect the things you are able to do which is good portion control, proper meal timing, healthy caloric intakes and healthy living. Do not let your fears amplify your perceived leap into living healthy.

Of course, telling you to make time is a lot easier said than done. Adjusting your schedule to eat healthy may involve waking up 20 minutes early to make breakfast or spending 10 extra minutes making your lunch before bed, or simply using your TV time to be more productive with your nutrition! These are achievable tasks. You may think dinner is the most daunting of all, especially since I am forbidding you to eat microwaved or frozen meals, but it truly isn't. After college I was introduced to the magic of a crockpot! Whoa boy! This invention was a blessing on my life! All I had to do was season my meat, chop my veggies and potatoes, add a bit of water, olive oil, and seasoning, turn the crock pot on low and head out to tackle my day. When I returned home, the smell of slow cooked meat flooded the hallways and stairwells and I'd feel like a cartoon, paralyzed and helplessly following the heavenly smell. This was perfect! No butler, no chef, no roommate to help with food; it was only me with my busy schedule of 9 graduate classes, coaching Ohio University's Women's and Field sprint team, working as a Graduate Assistant, training clients, working out, studying and interning at Mountain River Physical Therapy in Parkersburg, West Virginia. Not only was dinner prepared as soon as I walked through the door, but it was an easy clean up. After I graduated from the crockpot, I took on the cast iron skillet, and man-oh-man, life became a little sweeter. My dad taught me the beauty of the skillet and how to cook atop the stove as well as baking with my skillet. The main differences between the crockpot and the cast iron skillet is time and meal size. When I am making larger meals that I can eat from for an entire week, or a meal where I am entertaining a few folks, I choose my crockpot. When looking for a smaller meal that has a baked or simmered flavor, I choose my skillet. Below are a few recipes that frequent my kitchen in the crockpot and the cast iron skillet.

Crock Pot Recipes:

MOM'S POT ROAST

1 -2/3 LB Pot Roast

1 Can Campbell's Cream of Mushroom Soup (Reduced Sodium)

1 Can Campbell's French Onion Soup (Reduced Sodium)

2 Medium sized potatoes - cubed

1/2 medium sized onion - sliced

1 Large carrot - sliced

Pepper and Garlic

Place vegetables in bottom of Crock Pot.

Salt and pepper roast and place in Crock Pot on top of vegetables.

Pour contents of both cans of soup over meat.

Slow cook for 6 - 8 hours.

Remove meat and place on large serving plate.

Use slotted spoon and remove vegetables. Place on plate surrounding meat.

Pour gravy in separate bowl and enjoy your simple meal.

MOM'S CREAMY CHICKEN & MUSHROOMS

4 Skinless boneless chicken breast halves

1 1/2 cups sliced mushrooms

1 small onion sliced

1/8 tsp minced garlic

1 Can Campbell's Cream of Mushroom Soup (Reduced Sodium)

1/2 cup milk (fat free)

1/8 tsp pepper

In skillet, in 1 tsp olive oil, brown chicken on each side (approx. 2 mins. each side)

In separate bowl, mix together soup, milk garlic and pepper.

Place chicken in Crock Pot followed by onions.

Pour soup/milk mixture over chicken.

Slow cook for 6 - 8 hours.

Remove meat and place on large serving plate.

Use slotted spoon to retrieve onions and place onions on top of chicken.

Pour gravy in separate bowl and enjoy your meal with serving chicken and gravy over cooked brown rice.

Cast Iron Skillet Recipes:

DAD'S HIGH PROTEIN & GOOD FIBER – CHICKEN AND SHRIMP

Ingredients

2 Skinless chicken breasts or three skinless thighs or some combination thereof. I prefer thighs to breasts because they seem to have more flavor.

½ cup of apple juice or cider.

1 Red Bell Pepper and 1 Yellow Bell Pepper – both thinly sliced. Bell Peppers have a natural sweetness, we eat and taste with our sight as well. The different colors add a variety to not only your taste pallet but also to the pallet of your sight.

½ medium White Onion and ½ medium Red Onion – rough cut

1 cup of whole broccoli cut to your size preference. The fibrous stem adds good nutrition.

Salt, pepper, oregano, and Cajun seasonings to taste

3 Tablespoons of olive oil

1 cup of cooked frozen, deveined tail on shrimp. Shrimp should be the medium or large size.

Directions

Prepare your chicken 45 minutes before the rest of your meal. Drizzle both sides with white wine vinegar and Extra Virgin Olive Oil and let sit for 15 minutes. Add a pinch of salt, pepper, oregano, and Cajun seasonings over each piece of chicken. Cover and let sit for another 30 minutes.

Cut all vegetables. Thinly slice bell peppers

Thaw the shrimp in cool water, remove tail, drain and dry, place in a container and add a tablespoon of Frank's ® RedHot® sauce, place to the side and let it marinade.

Melt the oil in your cast iron skillet on high heat. When thoroughly melted turn the fire down to medium high heat.

Add the chicken mixture, cover the pan, and cook 5 minutes on each side. Be sure to move the chicken around so as not to burn.

Remove the top and cube the chicken while still in the pan and cut up the chicken while still in the pan in order to retain all of the juices.

Turn the heat to high and add the Apple Juice/cider and bring the mixture to a simmer. Add the vegetables, thoroughly stir then cover and simmer mixture for 6 minutes.

Remove the top and let simmer for another 2-4 minutes to slightly reduce/evaporate some of the liquid. Remove from the heat and stir in the shrimp.

You are all done. This recipe can be served alone or over rice. If I decide to add rice, I prefer brown rice for the slightly nutty flavor and the health benefits.

Bon A petit.

24-Hours

No matter how you dice, spin or cut it, we all have the same 24-hours. We all have different responsibilities to tend to within this timeframe, but what makes some better managers of their time than others? Your responsibilities may range from work, school, kids, marital duties, traveling, business, research, leisure, etc. The question is, what is your priority? Above, I gave you an excerpt of my schedule during graduate school, but I still took the time to train. Though building my career and attempting to maintain my finances as a grad student was important, without my health or happiness, none of that matters. In 2012, the average American spent 34 hours watching television on a weekly basis (Hinckley, Entertainment, 2012). Now in 2014, due to the influx of the

DVR phenomenon, the average American spends 5hrs/day watching TV (Hinckley, Entertainment, 2014)! So I ask you, what is your priority?

Nutrients: How They Operate In Your Body

The purpose of eating is to replace the nutrients and energy lost throughout the day due to energy expended by the body's maintenance, repair and growth (Brown, 2004). The foods you eat are composed of various combinations of proteins, carbohydrates, lipids (fats), water, vitamins and minerals; all of which support your body's makeup.

Every morsel of food you consume is broken down into macro (large) and micro (small) nutrients. Micronutrients are substances required within the body in trace amounts for development, functionality and disease prevention. Micronutrients are categorized as vitamins (complex organic compounds that are naturally present in foods and are needed only in very small amounts) and minerals (items whose purposes resemble that of vitamins but they are elements found on the periodic table i.e. calcium and iron). Naturally, micronutrients are found in the foods we eat, but, the degree that foods are processed have drastically decreased the amount of micronutrients we receive in our diets due to the methods of processing and preserving foods.

Because everything in our lives needs to happen immediately, we have become a "microwave society" and as previously mentioned, we want things to happen more quickly and easily now, than ever before. Our food now endures such an extreme level of processing that many micronutrients are cooked off or chemically burned off. This process placing us in a perpetual state of nutrient deficiency leading to supplement dependency Eating fewer processed foods like canned goods or microwavable meals and replacing them with fresh foods is referred to as eating 'closer to the ground'. Making this adjustment will drastically increase the level of micronutrients extracted from consumed food, inevitably leading towards more energy, less aches/pain, less sick time and a happier life.

There are isles and isles of cans, frozen dinners, snacks and instant treats in our grocery stores while in other countries, many of our guilty pleasures are banned from their markets due to poor nutrient quality and long term health concern. Some of these foods include ractopamine-tainted meat, flame retardant drinks such as Mountain Dew, processed foods containing artificial food coloring and dyes, arsenic laced chicken, Olestra/Olean, farm-raised salmon and many other products. Yes, it is easier to buy frozen or canned dinners in bulk and eat off them throughout the week, but we are sacrificing temporary comfort for long term health. It is OK to take a trip to the grocery store once a week to restock produce and fresh meats. Make the time to be a better you.

I had a client whose goal was to get his body to such a high degree physiologically that he could try out for the Pittsburgh Steelers. We sat down and created a plan that potentially could prepare him for try-outs in 2 years. Session after session there was little to no improvement. In his initial consultation, he told me he ate healthy and didn't need any nutritional advices as he spoke of steak, potatoes and vegetables as his favorite dinner, which he often ate. After diving more intensely into his nutrition, this man (sigh) was eating canned meats, canned potatoes, canned cereal, canned milk, canned everything! First, I had no idea cereal could be canned. Second, the realization of the sheer level of effect the quality of his nutrition had on his performance during practice amazed me.

After encouraging him to eat fresh produce, introducing him to meal/nutrient timing and a few other tricks up my sleeve, he quickly began to progress during sessions. The **quality** of your foods drastically impact your health; and in my opinion, it is equally as important as what you actually eat!

Here are a few tips when you are shopping at your market or grocery store:

- **Eat more fruits and veggies!** At every meal ½ of your plate should be fruits and vegetables, ¼ whole grain and ¼ lean protein with an added source of dairy at each meal (see image below).

- **Shop the perimeter of the grocery store.** For the most part, the outer ring of your local grocery store contains fresh produce such as meats, cheeses, milk, juices (not drinks), fruits, vegetables and grains.
- **Eat more whole produce foods.**

"A whole food comes from a seed that has all the nutrients it needs to grow the plant; it's a complete package. Think about the benefits of what [this new] package will do for your body. This is not the same as nutrients added in, as we see in so many food products."
-Jason White, PhD

- **Carefully read food labels.** Some food items may boast they are low in carbs, while they are actually high in fat, just as other labels may promote health by being low in fat, when again, they are high in carbohydrates. Later in this section you will calculate your specific caloric requirements and you will use this figure to help you understand on a quantitative level, how much you are eating.
- **Be mindful of sodium content and intake.** As a rule of thumb, the sodium content is considered high if the nutrition label reads a sodium content in milligrams (mg) that is higher than calories/serving. Stay away from these items.

I highly suggest visiting www.ChooseMyPlate.gov as this website contains a wealth of information to help you dig deeper into your individual journey to weight loss through the Trinity of Health and Wellness. The below image is the new food guide "pyramid" produced by the United States Government. This new guide to proper nutrition has evolved from the old pyramid to the plate you see below, which allows you to more easily visualize how to construct your plate.

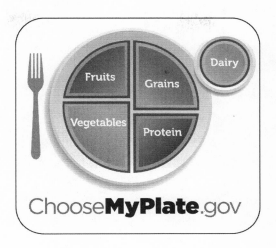

Vitamin Supplementation

By now you should be able to tell that I am huge proponent of eating "close to the ground". When you hear me say this, I am referring to eating things that have been through the least amount of processing possible. Choose fresh rather than frozen, stay away from cans as entrees, and if you feel you are fairly educated and you can't pronounce certain contents on the food label, chances are it's a processing agent. And do not, under any circumstances, purchase any full meals that have already been cooked that you have to thaw or microwave that are not from a health or weight loss company (I'm sure there are exceptions to this rule... but I don't know of any).

The fresher your food is, the more nutrient dense (higher amount of nutrients) it is causing you to get more bang for your buck. Does this mean that you *SHOULD NOT* be one of those individuals cramming your grocery cart(s) full of cans, microwave meals, Twinkies and Little Debby™ snack cakes? ABSOLUTELY!

Technically, any cooling mechanism is considered a preservative. You put your milk in the refrigerator to slow the buildup of bacteria and the aging process, therefore allowing it to last a bit longer. This is acceptable. In my grocery cart you will often see frozen fruit (for my summer smoothies), frozen fish (uncooked) and at times, frozen vegetables. All of these items have been frozen to stop the decomposition process that naturally occurs in organic items to keep them at their peak, but there are no added ingredients. Eating these foods and others such as chicken, shrimp, seafood etc. are acceptable to eat from frozen (as long as they are uncooked) as they still contain large amounts of healthy vitamins and minerals.

Many Americans struggle with getting adequate nutrients in their lifestyles due to the high amount of processed foods which are generally low in nutrient quality, and also very narrow personal food selections. Others may not receive proper nutrients due to absorption, utilization or production deficiencies, medications and available food options. With this said, these are the exceptions to the rule. If you are having trouble getting a wide and colorful array of fresh foods with the highest nutrient contents, then you may need to look at vitamin supplementation. Let me begin by saying protein is not a vitamin, and that there is only a very small population of people who actually need to protein supplement. Small children, adults 50 years and older, and elite athletes may protein supplement. Those transitioning from a processed life to "eating close to the ground", are suggested to take a multivitamin, along with those who may have issues absorbing or utilizing nutrients.

Do not get sucked into purchasing individual vitamin pills (Vitamin A, E, B complex, fish oil etc. unless suggested by a doctor), energy boosting packs, or anything with a Wham-Bam exciting name that promises a better sex life, more energy and longer hair. Many of these products are simply reimagined multivitamins or are packed full of nutrients your body can only utilize in small quantities. I call this Nutritional Marketing. Think about it, every one of these items on the shelf are created to grab your attention and scream, "Buy Me!" If a can of beans told you to jump off a cliff, would you? When comparing these labels to the labels of a multivitamin, you will find many of the same ingredients....vitamins and minerals. The label may also show that this particular product can increase your performance in bed *AND* wake you up the next morning to make a five course breakfast. The first thing that comes to my mind is high levels of vitamin B (again, just get it from your multivitamin).

A more important reason to stick with a multivitamin is that many other singular supplements (vitamin B, E, fish oil, flaxseed oil ect.) contain such high amounts of the substance that your body ends up passing most of the substance via urine or it may build up in the body setting the stage for future distress. Certain aspects of your body were designed to only use what it needs at that moment and the excess is discarded. When it comes to micronutrients and protein, your body can only use a certain amount, and after it has satisfied its quota, some particles just hang around in the body and the remaining becomes waste.

God made each body individually and uniquely; but in order to provide tips and advice based on facts, scientists created a standard regarding each micro and macronutrient determining, on average, the quantities that you should intake. This is referred to as the Recommended Daily Allowance (RDA). Again, as each body is unique, the individual requirements for various nutrients are different along with the suggested intake fluctuating throughout your lifespan. The RDA is a guideline based on age and gender that we should follow as not to over or under consume as either may cause a negative impact on your health. Scientists have also set a standard for the over consumption of each vitamin and mineral called the Tolerable Upper Intake Level (UL). For example, the accepted RDA for calcium is 1000mg/day. If you do not receive enough calcium in your daily lifestyle, early onset osteoporosis may occur, and in youth a calcium deficiency can drastically degrease and impair bone development making them more susceptible for osteoporosis later in life. Taking in too much calcium and continually surpassing the suggested UL of 2500mg/day can cause kidney stones, poor kidney function and it can hinder the proper absorption of other vitamins and minerals such as phosphorous, zinc and iron where if not absorbed can have devastating effects on the body's functionality. Consuming too much or too little of anything, as my mother would say, can kill you.

Everything you do will affect your body, but you have to be informed enough to be able to operate out of wisdom as opposed to ignorance. Again, my suggestion on vitamin supplementing is only for those who cannot receive proper nutrients from the food they consume. If you do decide to supplement, my suggestion is to take a multivitamin and only go outside of that suggestion if guided by a physician or nutritionist.

"My people are destroyed for the lack of knowledge: because thou hast rejected knowledge, I will also reject thee..."
-Hosea 4:6

Vitamins and Minerals

The scientific community presently accepts 13 vitamins which need to be consumed from food as they cannot be created within the body. Vitamins are essential to the growth, development and maintenance of the body at the cellular level.

Below is a chart of the 13 accepted vitamins along with information about what each vitamin is used for and general sources where that vitamin can be found.

Design Your Body Challenge

Fill your grocery cart with some of the above items that are outside of your normal shopping patterns. Purchase at least 7 items outside of your norm. If they are extremely unfamiliar to you, look up healthy recipes.
What are they?

_____
_____
_____
_____
_____

Vitamins

Vitamin	Food Sources	Functions
A	Liver, oranges, yellow fruits, leafy vegetables, carrots, pumpkin, squash, spinach, fish, soy milk and milk	Maintains epithelial membrane structures, resistance to infections and is necessary for the prevention of night blindness
B1 (Thiamine)	Pork, oatmeal, brown rice, most vegetables, potatoes liver and eggs	Carbohydrate metabolism, maintaining normal digestion and appetite, maintain nervous tissue function
B2 (Riboflavin)	Most dairy, banana, popcorn, green beans, asparagus	Formation of various enzymes and cellular oxidation, normal growth, production of red blood cells, health of skin, mucous membranes and eyes
B3 (Niacin)	Meats, fish, eggs, vegetables, mushrooms and nuts	Enhances nerve function, appetite and digestion, important in glycolysis, tissue respiration and fat synthesis
B5 (Pantothenic Acid)	Meat, broccoli and avocados	Aids in protein, fat and carbohydrate metabolism, assists in the formation of cholesterol and hormones
B6 (Pyridoxine)	Meat vegetables, nuts and bananas	Metabolizes tryptophan, needed for certain amino acid utilizations, aids in red blood cell formation, and nervous system function, healthy skin
B7 (Biotin)	Egg yolk, liver, peanuts, green leafy vegetables	A coenzyme in fatty acid and glycogen synthesis, assists in amino acid metabolism
B9 (Folic Acid)	Leafy vegetables, nuts and bananas	A coenzyme in the synthesis of nucleic acids and protein, normal function of hematopoietic system
B12 (Cyanocobalamin)	Animal products	Red blood cell formation, synthesis of nucleic acids
C (Ascorbic Acid)	Most fruits, vegetables and liver	Formation of cellular structures such as skin, dentin, cartilage, and bone, heals wounds and fractured bones, increases resistance to infections and facilitates iron absorption
D (Cholecalciferol)	Fish, eggs, liver, and mushrooms	Regulates the absorption of calcium and phosphorus from the intestinal tract
E (Alpha Tocopherol)	Most fruits, vegetables, nuts and seeds	Prevents damage to cellular membranes, maintains involuntary nervous, vascular and muscle systems
K (Phytomenadione)	Green leafy vegetables, purple vegetables, egg yolks, and liver	A coenzyme in fatty acid and glycogen synthesis, aids in blood clotting and bone formation

(Brown, 2004) (ExRx.net, 2014)

Because our lifestyle mainly consists of processed foods and we no longer eat "close to the ground", many Americans find themselves deficient in certain vitamins. Many vitamin deficiencies or even overdoses may cause diseases or other adverse symptoms.

Dietary minerals are also required by the body, but separately from vitamins, they are naturally occurring elements that present themselves on the Periodic Table. These elements are needed in trace amounts, so much so that some elements such as Boron have a role, but scientists cannot detect at what level this role is played and therefore do not have an RDA. As many as 26 elements are required in order for the body to function and below are the few that have been studied and length.

Minerals

Mineral	Food Source	Functions
Calcium	Milk and dairy products, dark leafy vegetables	Bone and teeth formation, nerve and muscle function, blood clotting
Chloride	Salt	Nerve and muscle function, water balance
Chromium	Meats, black pepper, green pepper, potato, spinach, parsnips, fresh chili, carrots, apple, banana, orange, blueberries, cheese, egg, beans, grains	Glucose metabolism by increasing the effects of insulin. Assists in protein, carbohydrate and fat metabolism.
Copper	Meat, poultry, liver, seafood, fish, oysters, green vegetables, whole grains, legumes, peas	Formation of red blood cells, maintains health of bones, blood vessels, nerve and immune systems
Fluoride	Fish, seafood, milk, tea	Bone and teeth growth
Iodine	Saltwater seafood, seaweed, dairy, whole-grain cereal	Thyroid hormone formation
Iron	Red meat, liver, kidney, shellfish, egg yolks, beans, leafy green vegetables, apricots, whole grains	O2 transport in red blood cells, production of hemoglobin and myoglobin, enzyme function, assists in thyroid hormone synthesis
Magnesium	Raw dark leafy greens, nuts, beans, soybeans/soy products, whole grains, fish, crab, oysters, scallops, kelp, potato, sweet potato, beets, avocado, figs, apricots, dates, prunes, raisins, banana, blackberry, coconut	Essential to bone growth and cell production, regulates neuromuscular sensitivity
Manganese	Leafy greens, vegetables, nuts, beans, whole grains, fruits, tea	Enzymatic function
Molybdenum	Whole grains, eggs, meat, poultry, fish, crab, organ meats, peas, beans, cauliflower, spinach, garlic	Energy metabolism

Phosphorus	Milk and dairy products, egg yolks, meat, poultry, fish, whole grains, beans, peas, soybeans	Bone teeth and membrane formation, maintains body's proper acid/base balance and nerve/muscle function
Potassium	Bananas, citrus fruits, fresh vegetables, potatoes, legumes, whole grains, milk and dairy, meats, fish, nuts, seeds	Regulates fluid balance, nerve impulse transmission, muscle contraction and heart and kidney function
Selenium	Beef, chicken, lamb, turkey, beef liver, scallops, clams, oysters, crab, lobster, shrimp, herring, smelt, cod, tuna, halibut, salmon, egg yolks, dairy products, whole grains, crimini mushrooms, onions, and garlic	Prevention of fat and body chemical breakdown, cellular defense system for antioxidants, thyroid hormone synthesis and metabolism, protects the thyroid gland from damage via excessive iodine exposure
Sodium	Table salt, dairy products, processed foods	Nerve and muscle function, fluid balance
Zinc	Beef, chicken, liver, seafood, dairy products, eggs, whole grains, legumes, peas, nuts	Required to produce enzymes necessary for digestion, cell division, growth and repair (healing), helps immune system function properly, assists in taste and smell acuity

(Brown, 2004) (ExRx.net, 2014)

The All Mighty Calorie:

As mentioned earlier, when you eat, each morsel of food is broken down into carbohydrates, proteins, lipids (fats), vitamins, minerals and water, but calories only come from the breakdown of proteins, carbohydrates (carbs) and lipids.

A calorie is a single unit of energy measured by its ability to raise 1 gram of water 1°C. Macronutrients are the nutrients that your body needs in large quantities due to their ability to generate calories. Macronutrients include protein, carbohydrates and fats which are broken down to be used as energy. Carbohydrates, fats and protein should be consumed in specific quantities based on age, height, weight, gender and activity level. Everything you eat is broken down and categorized as a carbohydrate (glucose or sugar), a fat (triglycerides or free fatty acids), or a protein (amino acids, both essential and non-essential). There are optimal percentages of each macronutrient that are recommended to satisfy various physiological requirements and assist you through the stages of your life. For example, a teenager is going to require more total calories from carbs than is an individual trying to lose weight; just as a professional athlete will have a higher caloric intake and higher percentages of carbs and protein than what is necessary for you in your weight loss journey.

Unlike micronutrients, macronutrients present calories for the body. Calories are the body's main source of fuel, much like the fuel of a car. Unlike a car, your body never turns off and is always active and always requiring energy even during sleep (Brown, 2004), but this does not mean you should be constantly eating. About 60% of calories used by the body are used solely for maintaining vital functions such as body temperature, respiration rates, heartbeat, and cell functions. About 10% is used for digestion and nutrient absorption, and the remaining 30% is required to replace the calories burned by our daily physical activity (Brown, 2004).

The problem is that we consume more calories than what is needed to replace the calories burned from daily activity leaving us in a positive caloric balance. Because we have overeaten, our bodies store this excess pool of calories/energy as fat and tuck them away in fat deposits creating lovely curves that most of us are dying to get rid of. It is important to note that not all macronutrients can be stored, only carbohydrates and fats. Excess protein is excreted from the body, along with other micronutrients in excess that the body cannot use. Due to our habits of eating in excess, Americans are said to have some of the richest urine in the world as the urine is packed full of micronutrients and amino acids (components of proteins) due to constant overconsumption.

Have you ever noticed that certain foods make you fuller faster (satiety factor; how full you feel), or that your body responds differently than normal? You may even joke about how certain foods go right to your trouble areas. This can be due to the individual energy yield of each macronutrient and its satiety factor. In every gram of carbohydrates you eat, four calories are gleaned for energy (4cals/g). Protein follows suit with carbs, as one gram of protein yields 4cals (4cals/g); while fat more than doubles the energy yield of carbs and proteins. Consuming one gram of fat yields 9 calories (9cals/g)! Alcohol is another energy-producing compound that yields 7 calories per gram (7cals/g). With this said, people who complain of contracting the "beer belly" disease, are actually telling the truth. Yes, the only way to gain energy is by consuming calories, but remember excess calories are what is converted and stored as fat cells or glucose within the body.

Remember, your body requires energy/calories to operate as calories act as the energy currency of the body. For every action/function your body is engaged in, whether consciously or unconsciously, energy is required. Unconsciously, your body requires energy for temperature regulation, heart rate control, digestion, cell functions, muscle and tissue function and support, growth, regeneration etc. Consciously, energy is needed for physical activity, regulating stress levels, laughing, crying, etc. Because of this, there is a specific number of calories you should be consuming, on a daily basis, built on your physiological status and the energy requirements of your body.

Scientists have discovered a way to calculate the number of calories your body requires to function on a day to day basis. You can generally search for the term "caloric requirement calculator" but I prefer the American Council on Exercise's Daily Caloric Needs Estimator. Follow this link, add your age, height, gender and activity level, and the estimator will compute a figure which indicates how many calories you should be consuming in order to maintain your current weight. As you continue to lose weight, revisit this calculator after every stent of 10lb weight loss as your caloric requirements will change as your weight decreases.

http://www.acefitness.org/acefit/healthy
living_tools_content.aspx?id=4

My estimated caloric requirement is: _____ Date: _____

One of the most helpful tips I can give to assist you in your weight loss journey is related to your nutrition. Though there is currently no true way to scientifically quantify the importance of nutrition in relation to cardiovascular exercise or resistance training, just know it is extremely important. After discovering your estimated caloric requirement, you now have the ability to act on and adjust your eating by basing it on caloric balance as discussed above.

You should understand the equation, calories in vs. calories out. Again, if you take in too many calories and too few are burned through daily activity (conscious and unconscious), those calories will be stored in the body as fat or carbohydrates. Opposing this, if you burn more calories than what you intake, you move your body into a state of weight loss. Unless otherwise indicated, each caloric requirement calculator will give you a figure that represents the calories needed to maintain your current weight which is equivalent to calories in = calories out. Since the crux of this book is about weight loss, I assume you do not want to maintain your current weight. Below is an extremely important fact to assist with weight loss via nutrition, and how to numerically adjust the equation calories in = calories out.

In order to move to a state of negative caloric balance (calories in < calories out) and weight loss via nutrition, reduce your daily caloric intake by 500 calories per day to lose 1lb of fat per week, or by 1000 calories per day to lose up to 2lbs of fat per week.

NOTE: You should *NOT* restrict yourself to consuming less than 1000 calories/day as this becomes unhealthy and can actually cause you to gain weight due to the chain reactions that occur when your body enters a state of starvation. It is best to lose weight by combining both caloric reduction via nutrition and increasing calories burned/out with exercise. Nutrition alone will only get you so far. Calories restricted from diet, plus calories burned from exercise increase the total number of calories out. When calories out > calories in, you have entered a state of negative energy balance and in a state of weight loss. BOOM.

Popup Coach: View this website for a quick description of calories entitled, "Calories, How Much is Too Much?" https://www.youtube.com/watch?v=077bTx6mt44

1 Pound of Fat

There is a specific reason why the recommended caloric reduction is 500-1000cals/day. If for seven days, you reduce your caloric intake by 500cals, you will lose 1lb of fat in that 7 day period. Just the same, reducing your caloric intake by 1000cals/day will cause you to lose 2lbs of fat in that seven day period.

One pound of fat is equivalent to 3,500 calories. Therefore, when your weight scale is consistently 1lb higher than in previous weeks, it is likely that your calories in for that past week was 3,500cals greater than your calories out.

It is my recommendation to reduce your daily caloric intake by 500cals/day and increase your calories out by burning 200-500cals via exercise per day. Together, the caloric reductions from both diet and exercise are equivalent to 700-1000cals/day which can be added to your calories in vs. calories out equation.

Equally as important, it takes 2,500cals to build 1lb of muscle. In order to build muscle your body must be in a state of positive caloric balance. This means that calories in ≥ calories out. But muscle building cannot be accomplished by cardio alone. If you are overweight, you have been in a positive caloric balance for quite some time where very little (if any) muscle was gained; you may have just as easily lost muscle mass which was replaced with fat mass. In order to build muscle you must have adequate sources of protein and carbs which gives your body the right tools or building blocks to build muscle, but you must also lift weights with vigor and intensity. Lifting weights for strength, size or endurance gives your body the bricks and mortar it needs to build with. Muscle building will be further explained in chapter 8. Without proper weight training, your positive caloric balance will become fat gain.

Weight Check:

My current weight is: _____lbs x 2.2lbs/kg is: _____ kg, Today's date: _____

My waist circumference is: _____inches, Today's date: _____

My hip circumference is: _____inches, Today's date: _____

Let's consider Jessica:

Jessica is a 32 year old accountant weighing 193lbs, 5'7", has a BMI of 30.3 and is extremely sedentary, but has been wondering why she has steadily picked up weight over the past few years. Jessica has set her weight loss goal to 34lbs of fat which will bring her BMI down to 24.9 putting her in the "normal" weight category for her height. After determining her caloric requirement based on the link provided above, she has determined that the max amount of calories she should be consuming is 1943cals/day and her sodium intake is almost triple the acceptable range. Her normal caloric intake is usually closer to 2800cals/day as she never eats breakfast, always eats out at fast food chains for lunch and her dinners typically consist of reheating freezer meals. On average, Jessica has been eating 857cals/day over the caloric requirement for a sedentary woman of her and her stature. This answers her question of why she has been steadily gaining almost 2lbs/week!

Her first step is to start cutting calories by eating what is required by her body and not over eating by 857 calories. In order to re-acclimate her system to eating 1943cals/day, Jessica must begin to eat more frequently throughout the day. The goal is to eat 5-6times per day. I suggest 3 small meals and 3 large snacks, 3 hours between each. This means that Jessica needs to consume foods closer to this schedule:

- a small breakfast at 7am (oatmeal and fruit),
- a large pre-lunch snack at 10am (PB&J),
- a small lunch at 1pm (medium salad and fruit),
- a large pre-dinner snack at 4pm (granola bar and finger veggies),

- a small dinner at 7pm (broccoli, fish and a sweet potato), and
- a small post-dinner snack at 10pm (fruit or veggies).

Jessica has now learned how to prepare her meals for the next day and even a few days out, allowing her to attain 5-6 meals/day and reach her target caloric intake of 1943cals/day. Now, Jessica has lost a few pounds

> Did you know that if you skip breakfast you are 4 times more likely to become obese?

simply by reducing her overeating, to the amount of calories that she should be eating. Jessica is now ready to take it to the next step.

Because of Jessica's schedule, she feels she doesn't have enough time to exercise just yet, but she has continued her weight loss journey by reducing her required daily calories of 1943 by 500cals/day. After a few weeks, Jessica has seen a steady 1lb decrease in weight and is excited about the possibilities of increasing fat loss that she can get from adding exercise to her schedule. She has decided to wake up 30 minutes early each day to go for a brisk morning walk to increase her calories burned adding to her calories out. Though she only walks 30 minutes, the higher the intensity she walks (intensity can be varied by speed, hills, adding jogging, adding hand weights or anything to make that 30mins of activity harder), the more calories she can burn. More specific details on intensity can be found in Chapter 6.

Protein

Proteins are large molecules composed of long chains of amino acids and are the building blocks of the body as they control vast amounts of biological functions from cellular structures to whole body locomotion. One gram of protein provides your body with 4calories worth of energy. Though we know protein to be most famous for muscle building, it also plays a vital role in the formation of the brain, nervous system, blood, skin and hair, along with assisting in the transportation of iron, vitamins, minerals, fat and oxygen. Protein also assists in maintaining the acid-base and fluid balances of the body.

There are 20 known amino acids, 8-10 of which can be manufactured within the body while the remainder are essential amino acids that must be absorbed from the foods we eat. Amino acids are found within many substances that we eat but the only products considered to be complete proteins are those which contain the 10-12 amino acids that cannot be found within the body. Animal products are complete proteins as they contain all essential amino acid. Proteins in plant foods usually do not contain all essential amino acids and therefore are considered incomplete proteins. One main exception to this rule is soy which is a plant based complete protein. As plant based foods are considered incomplete proteins, individuals who do not eat meat or meat products must gain their daily protein by combining incomplete proteins in hopes to satisfy the body's requirements for complete proteins. This is achieved by pairing incomplete proteins such as rice and beans to create a complete protein as the essential amino acids in rice pair with the essential amino acids in beans. This process is called protein complementarity.

Though protein provides 4cals/g, it is not the preferred or primary source of energy as very little protein is used for fuel. If carbs are not sufficiently provided, the existing protein (muscles, amino acids and cell tissue) can be converted into glucose through the process of gluconeogenesis. If your body enters a gluconeogenic state by using existing resources, your body has become catabolic and begins to eat itself (no Bueno). When the body does not receive enough carbs and therefore glucose due to extremely low caloric intakes or low carb diets, it begins to enter a starvation state. In this starvation state, your body shifts to survival mode and not only converts existing resources into usable energy, but it also holds fast to the fat and carbs that are consumed making it harder to lose weight. Each individual has a baseline level of the amount of carbs that they should intake. The general recommendation is not to go below 1,000cals/day but it is my belief that once going below your Basal Metabolic Rate (the amount of calories your body, organs, tissues and functions need to survive during 24 hours of absolutely no activity), your body begins the process of triggering this starvation state.

Above all, your body will protect the brain which is only fed by glucose through the blood. Have you noticed times where you were extremely hungry and you developed a slight head ache or dizziness? This is your brain telling you that its resources are growing low and it needs to be fed. After a short period of time, you may have noticed that your headache or dizziness has dissipated. The liver has released extra stores of glucose into the blood stream to travel to the brain and other tissue to be used as energy. This is your body's last ditch effort before it enters the catabolic state of gluconeogenesis (remember this is the state where your body begins to break down muscle to use for energy) (Austrailian Bureau of Statistics/Commonwealth Department of Health and Ageing., 1998).

In order to build muscle, you must be in an anabolic state, which allows your body to create larger molecules from smaller products. Being in this state of anabolism allows muscle to be made or built from amino acids and proteins. Here we are looking to create the environment of protein synthesis. When most individuals think of beginning a muscle building nutrition program, their mind immediately jumps to a high protein and low carb diet. What most individuals aren't aware of is the fact that if a sufficient number of carbs aren't present in the diet, protein synthesis cannot occur, therefore muscle cannot be built without carbs.

The RDA of protein is 0.8g/kg/day for the average individual. Remember, divide your current weight in pounds by 2.2kg, then multiply that figure by 0.8g. Ex: Nate weights 286lbs/2.2kg = 130kg. 130kg X 0.8g of pro = 104g of pro/day.

Find your protein intake: _____

A study done by Skov, et al., found that obese individuals eating a higher protein diet (25% of total calories from protein) lost significantly more weight and body fat than those eating a lower protein diet (12%

of total calories from protein). My recommendation to you is to have a protein intake of 25-30% of your caloric intake. The danger with protein is that most animal and meat products tend to contain high levels of saturated fat. When engaging in increasing your current protein intake, take heed to only consuming lean meats. Meats are usually marked with the percentage of lean meat to fat; try your best to find lean meats that are 90% lean and above (80% lean is a bare minimum). Concerning chicken and pork, I have found the quality of meat usually depends upon the brand. Cut the fat off lower quality meats and enjoy. Regarding fish and seafood, wild is better than farm raised. In pigmented fish like tuna and salmon, you can see the marbling or striations of fat just as you would in uncooked red meats, choose the options which have the least amounts of visible marbling. The best sources of complete protein are eggs, milk, fish and meat while the incomplete proteins in beans, lentils, peas, and peanuts can be combined with whole grains, brown rice, corn, nuts and/or seeds to create complete proteins (Skov, Toubro, Holm, & Astrup, 1999).

Consuming protein and carbs surrounding workouts provides your body with the energy (from calories) necessary to push through the workout, along with creating a readily available source of protein for muscle repair and carbs for energy post-workout. Once you have reached the stage of major muscle building, I suggest consuming some form of protein and carbs (chicken, fish or supplement) 45 mins before your workout and within 45 mins post workout. When consuming large amounts of protein it is important to maintain water intake 2oz per pound of body weight as protein intake can cause dehydration.

The Dreaded Carbohydrate!

Some diets suggest carbs are evil and that you should consume protein in larger quantities than carbohydrates including fruits/vegetables. Well, I disagree. Carbohydrates are a required source of nutrition granting you the biggest "bang for your buck" in healthy energy creation.

Carbohydrates are the body's main and preferred source of energy, though energy can be created from both fat and protein. It is true that carbs hold water which can cause your body to hold extra water weight. But again, the important aspects of nutrition are quantity and quality. Forty-five to 65% of your daily energy intake should be derived from carbs. Though this number seems high, and carbs are made out to be evil, your body thrives within this range. I would suggest sticking to 45-55% carbs for your daily intake and stay away from the higher range in this number due to your goals of weight loss.

Remember that all meats provide protein, all oils, margarines, and meats will give you fats, and guess what; everything else breaks down into carbs. This means that vegetables, fruits, pasta, rice, legumes, sugar, and some starches are considered carbs. Many people end up eating above their suggested range of 45-65% carbs even if they may not consume large quantities of food on a daily basis because they may not be aware of how the food is digested and broken down once consumed.

Consuming more than my suggested range of carbs (45-55% of total caloric intake) causes you to run the risk of increasing total calories in, as calories out remain the same which increases the potential for a positive caloric balance and therefore weight gain. Large intakes of carbs can also increase triglyceride levels as carbs can be converted and stored as fat, and it inevitably increases body fat by repressing fat oxidation. Equally, consuming too few carbs has an interesting compellation of reactions. If you decrease the total amount of carbs you consume, your body is forced to use fat as its primary energy source. Sounds good right? The side effects to this energy usage are: endurance can be reduced up to 50%, glycogen stores are depleted, and ketogenesis begins. Ketogenesis is the creation of ketone bodies when glycogen stores are depleted, again, entering the starvation state. When ketone bodies are used for energy you may experience the symptoms of weakness, dizziness, tunnel vision, fatigue and bad breath (ketoacidosis). For diabetics this is extremely dangerous as there is already an issue and inconsistency in getting glucose into the cell body, and eating a low carb diet has the potential to exacerbate the symptoms of diabetes along with unconsciousness, coma and possibly death. As stated above, in this situation blood glucose is maintained by gluconeogenesis (the breaking down of protein to create glucose). If a low carb diet is coupled with inadequate protein intake, protein from lean muscle and tissue will continue to be metabolized (ExRx.net, 2014), meaning that you are breaking down your existing tissue to feed itself.

Simple Sugars

Humans cannot produce carbohydrates which are a byproduct of plant photosynthesis. Therefore, we must consume plants in order to retrieve carbs from the diet by metabolizing plants. Simple carbs (or simple sugars) are composed of either mono-(one), di-(two) or poly (many) saccharides (a unit of sugar) such as glucose, fructose or galactose. You are most likely familiar with glucose as it is the most common sugar. Glucose is the building block of all other carbohydrates, and is the substance that humans derive the most energy from. Fructose is commonly referred to as fruit sugar and is the sweetest of all saccharides (simple sugars).

Fructose is found in honey and high-fructose corn syrup in fruit flavored drinks and pops (yes, I am from the Mid-West!). Note that anything that says, "Drink", is artificially flavored and is not a true product of fruit. High-fructose items have been a hot topic as research as shown that as the use of high-fructose corn syrup has increased, so have the country's obesity levels (Nelson, R.D., L.D., 2012). Research has also proven that this substance is chemically similar to table sugar, so the question is whether the substance has assisted with the growing obesity epidemic in America, or is the cause related to higher sugar and fat intake in general. High-fructose corn syrup has yet to be identified as any less healthy than other types of sweeteners. Though this is true, high intakes of any type of sugar can contribute towards unwanted calories that are linked to health problems including weight gain, type 2 diabetes, metabolic syndrome and high triglyceride levels inevitably increasing your risk of heart disease (Nelson, R.D., L.D., 2012).

Galactose is rarely found freely occurring in nature but when it combines with glucose, it forms the disaccharide lactose which is the principal sugar found in milk. People who are lactose intolerant do not have the necessary enzyme (lactase) to breakdown the chemical bond between glucose and galactose, therefore causing lactose to become indigestible and causes digestive issues and discomfort. Sucrose and maltose are also disaccharides along with lactose. Sucrose is found in sugar cane, sugar beets and table sugar (white, brown or powdered sugar). Maltose (malt sugar) is produced from the chemical decomposition of starches.

Simple sugars are fast digesting and produce fast and high blood sugar spikes. Beware of over consuming simple sugars as these blood sugar spikes negatively affect your metabolism by creating drastic peaks and valleys instead of a consistent stream of energy.

Complex Carbohydrates

Polysaccharides are long chain sugar molecules and are considered to be complex carbohydrates. Starch, glycogen and fiber are the most important polysaccharides in our diet. Starch is a digestible long chain carbohydrate and is typically found in the seeds of plants which is where plant energy is stored. If you remember back to high school chemistry, you were taught that energy is created or absorbed by breaking bonds (the things that hold molecules together to form new stuff); when the bonds of disaccharides and polysaccharides are broken via enzymatic action, energy is released. Now that these long chain molecules have been broken, glucose is free to be used for energy production by way of being absorbed into the blood stream (or to be stored in the muscle or liver as glycogen).

Glycogen, which is a long chain animal carbohydrate (found in animals and seafood), and starch, a long chain plant carbohydrate found in grains and vegetables, are considered complex carbohydrates. Due to the manner that meat is brought to your table, most glycogen in animal products is depleted before you are able to consume it, therefore the majority of consumable glycogen is consumed through plants. Because starch and glycogen have longer chain compilations, they take longer to digest and also require more energy to complete the process of digestion. This is the positive factor of eating complex carbohydrates, due to the increased amount of energy that is required to process the meal, along with the increased time it takes to degest. This keeps your metabolism steadier for longer periods of time. In short, complex carbohydrates burn more calories to process and present themselves strongest in whole grains.

Popup Coach: Remember, diets are temporary and lifestyle changes are forever. I will refer to the word "diet" it two forms, one as the structure and content of what you typically consume, and two if you are on a quick diet for a short season. Example, when I train for a photo shoot, vacation or a special event, I will put myself on a diet for the purpose of weight loss with a caloric restriction/expenditure (inclusive of both diet and exercise combined) of 500-800cals/day. Unless you only plan to diet for a season, remove this word from your vocabulary. The thing you should focus on with your lifestyle change is an adjustment of portion control. Check out this video "Diet vs Portion Control" for hints, tips and advice https://www.youtube.com/watch?v=sYpwo5NfiUI.

Glycemic Index

The Glycemic Index (GI) is a system used to rate and categorize the rise in blood glucose following consuming a particular food. The GI categorizes food as high, medium or low based on the measured rises in blood glucose as compared to white bread (an extremely high GI food due to the sugar content). Factors that affect the GI rating are ripeness, cooking, protein, fat content, and handling, causing the GI categorization of many foods to be very. The GI rating does not indicate the relative health of that food item, it only determines blood sugar rises which can be used for different purposes difficult (for example, ice-cream is a low GI food due to its large fat content). For example; when I competed in Division I Track and Field for the University of Dayton, about 45mins before I competed in an event like the 100 Hurdles or the 200 meter dash, I'd eat a plain white bagel (extremely high on the GI scale), and about 10-15 minutes before the race, I'd eat gummy treats (almost pure sugar). This spiked my blood sugar levels providing me with the necessary boost of natural energy my system needed to pull out a win. Lower GI foods take longer to digest, require more energy for digestion and they keep you feeling fuller longer as there is no drastic drop or crash in blood sugar which often makes you feel drained of energy and/or feeling hungry. Your goal is to shoot for low GI foods that are good nutritious choices.

A small representation of the Glycemic Index

High GI ≥ 70	Medium GI 56-69	Low GI ≤ 55
White Bread	Rye Bread	Pumpernickel Bread
Corn Flakes	Refined Pasta	Oatmeal
Dried Fruit	Ice Cream	Plain yogurt
Instant White Rice	Blueberries	Strawberries

For a full review of the GI, visit http://www.glycemicindex.com/

The question of carbohydrates now becomes, "which type of carbohydrate is better for me and my weight loss?" My suggestion is to lean towards medium to low GI foods as they will not cause your blood glucose to spike after consumption which is dangerous for diabetics, and it is another source of caloric expenditure allowing you to burn a few more calories.

Keeping a level blood sugar is important as:

- It keeps your metabolism functioning steadily throughout the day (as opposed to peaks and valleys where it is over worked then underutilized)

- If blood sugar is rapidly increased, insulin levels will also rapidly increase leading to an increase in accumulating fat deposits (ACE - American Council on Exercise, 2011, p. 190)
- A link exists between the GI and weight loss where scientist have found an inverse relationship between the intake of sugary carb-loaded foods and obesity - The higher up the food is on the GI scale, the more likely you are to gain weight.
- Blood glucose spikes may lead to overeating and consequent weight gain
- Consuming low GI foods may lead to a significant decrease in low-density lipoproteins (LDLs also known as bad cholesterol).
- Though some research is sketchy, it majorly shows that a high carb and high protein diet while keeping foods in the low GI range can assist in providing significant weight loss, particularly fat mass.

The Glycemic Load is also used as a measure of blood sugar rises specifically for carbs that are combined with other substances such as proteins or fats (as the presence of these macronutrients change the glycemic "blood sugar" effect). The Glycemic Load is measured by multiplying the GI food by the total number of carbs (g), divided by 100.

Glycemic load = GI x carbs (g)/100. The glycemic load is used to indicate how much a given amount of food will affect blood sugar levels.

Why is maintaining a steady metabolism so important? Anytime you eat your body begins to digest and absorb the food you ate to be used as energy. Digestion begins as soon as food hits your mouth and continues on through your stomach and the three different areas of your digestive tract. As food is broken down into macro and micronutrients, glucose is released and absorbed into the blood stream in high amounts. The content and amount of carbs you consumed dictates how much glucose (sugar) enters your blood at one time. The glucose in your blood then gets absorbed into cells (by the action of insulin) to be further broken down (via glycolysis, the process of breaking down glucose) to become and be used as pure energy. Blood glucose levels become extremely high due to ingesting simple carbohydrates (which are typically high GI food). When these levels become elevated (hyperglycemia), the body releases a surge of insulin, which again, acts as the key to open the doors of cells to use glucose as energy. This point of elevated blood sugar and insulin is typically where your body feels wired or excited. This is due to large amounts of glucose entering the cell and being created into energy for immediate use. The subsequent crash after this high occurs when the increased flow of insulin has caused too much glucose to be absorbed into the cell and the remaining blood glucose has reached dangerously low levels (hypoglycemia) which drastically decreases the flow of energy into the cell. On the light end, hypoglycemia can cause you to feel sluggish, headaches, drained and just... "Blah". The dangers of hypoglycemia can be life threatening as you may experience seizures and nervous system damage.

Referring back to metabolism, every time you eat you will inevitably have a rise in blood glucose. During the time blood glucose levels have fallen due to the actions of insulin (remember glucose gets absorbed into cells to be used as energy because insulin is the key that unlocks the cell door), your metabolism (the system that burns resources to create energy) slows down. It is true, some people have higher/faster metabolisms than others but the goal is to keep blood glucose levels as steady as possible to keep your metabolism moving and constantly burning fuel. One way to keep your metabolism steadily moving and burning energy is to consume low GI and low glycemic load foods, and to eat on a timed schedule. Your body can easily break down simple carbs, which again, causes the almost immediate spike in blood sugar, while it takes a longer time for the body to digest complex carbs due to their structure of long chains. As the body cleaves resources from the long chain/complex carbohydrates, the separated glucose molecules are absorbed and used as energy, while portions of the complex carb have not yet been absorbed. This causes an extended digestion and consequently an extended absorption keeping blood glucose levels more steady and allowing your metabolism to operate on a continuous basis.

Fiber

Fiber is found in the category of complex carbohydrates as its sources are found in all plant-based foods. Though fiber is a substance that cannot be directly used for energy, it is an essential aspect of good health. Those who live fiber rich lifestyles see the benefits of lower cholesterol and a reduced risk of CVD and diabetes. Generally, Americans tend to live low fiber lifestyles and only consuming 12-15g/d while the RDA is 20-35g. Consuming higher amounts of fiber within the range of 40-50g/d may cause gas and it is suggested to increase your fluid intake (ExRx.net, 2014).

Diets high in fiber have been proven to provide health benefits such as a healthy gastrointestinal tract, lower risk of colon cancer, low cholesterol, it helps prevent constipation, hemorrhoids and many people who maintain a lifestyle rich in fiber often carry less fat than the average individual who does not. There are two types of fiber; soluble/digestible fiber which has the ability to dissolve in water and therefore digested, while insoluble/indigestible fiber does not dissolve in water and cannot be digested. Though it possesses no caloric content, insoluble fiber assists your digestive tract in providing mass to ease and speed the movement of waste through your intestines. Soluble fibers, also known as dietary fiber, slow the absorption of glucose into the blood stream and has a longer digestion time as its chemical makeup takes longer to breakdown. An increased digestive time keeps you fuller longer leading towards a lower level of hunger combating obesity and overeating. They also specifically help reduce blood cholesterol, and therefore heart disease and atherosclerosis.

As an easy reference, insoluble/indigestible fibers help to increase satiety and decrease caloric intake. Therefore, the more insoluble fiber you ingest, not only are you cleansing your gastrointestinal tract, but you are consuming less total calories even if you do not change to total amount of food eaten in that meal.

Sweeteners

Noncaloric sweeteners are calorie free because your body cannot metabolize them and they are used to add that familiar sweet taste to foods and beverages. Aspartame (also known as Equal®, NutraSweet®, Sunett®, and sweet One®) are approved for use in the United States, though early studies discovered that they may be linked to causing bladder cancer in laboratory rats. This has caused a sizeable scare amongst the health community though scientists have not found the same effect in humans. As I've stated before, just eat "close to the ground". Try honey if you need an added source of sugar.

Fats

Fat; the very word makes some cringe and others sneer. Truth be told, the over consumption of fat isn't the main reason you are overweight, the over consumption of carbohydrates is the culprit. All macronutrients are essential to the body, including fat as it serves many purposes and are the most abundant form of energy within the body. Fats contain 9cals/g which is 225% more calories than both carbs and protein (4carbs/g each) (ACE - American Council on Exercise, 2011). Because fats are the most calorie dense, you must be mindful of the amount consumed as weight loss and weight control is the goal.

To begin this section, let's focus on the positive attributes of this macronutrient. Fats have many uses in the body such as energy storage, insulation, nerve transmission, hormone production, assistance with the formation of cellular membrane structures, and the essential fatty acids lenolenic and lenoleic assist with brain development, inflammation control, and blood clotting. Fat is also the only substance that can absorb vitamins A, D, E, and K.

Monounsaturated fatty acids are heart healthy fats. Monounsaturated fats are Omega-9 fatty acids that can be identified as being liquid at room temperature due to possessing one double bond that connects two carbon atoms together while missing 2 hydrogen atoms (too sciency? I know, but it will be an important identifier in a few). This double bond causes a kink or bend in its structure inhibiting it from holding a true form, causing monounsaturated fatty acids (MUFAs) to be liquid at room temperature. Omega-9 is the most common MUFA found in foods and is commonly found in olive, canola and peanut oil, nuts, peanut butter, seeds, avocados, olives, meats and whole milk. These fats are considered heart healthy as they have the potential to lower low density lipoproteins (LDL) which is considered "bad cholesterol" while maintaining high density lipoprotein (HDL) levels, which are reversely found as "good cholesterol" as it helps keep the heart healthy.

Very similar to MUFAs, polyunsaturated fatty acids (PUFAs) are liquid at room temperature and contain two or more double bonds connecting carbon atoms but they are missing four or more hydrogen atoms. Lenolenic acid (Omega-3) and linoleic acid (Omega-6) are PUFAs and regarded as essential to acquire within the food consumed as our bodies cannot synthesize them. Polyunsaturated fatty acids are more prone to oxidation which changes how your body reacts to these acids. Omega-3 fatty acids have earned their name due to the position of the first double bond in its carbon chain. Omega-3s, again also referred to as lenolenic acid, and its benefits include, but are not limited to:

- Maintaining cardiovascular health,
- Reducing triglyceride levels within the body,
- Holing importance in the prevention of rheumatoid arthritis, cancer and heart disease,
- Joint lubrication,
- Maintenance of mental clarity and
- Possesses anti-inflammatory properties.

Omega-3 fatty acids can be found in lake trout, herring, sardines, albacore tuna, cod, salmon, halibut, mahi-mahi, catfish, flounder, tilapia, bluefish and whitefish and has an intake recommendation of 7-11g/week.

Though there are positive attributes to the Omega-3 PUFA, it is recommended to limit your intake of fatty fish to 12oz (340g)/week. Many of the above fish also contain harmful chemicals and mercury whose intake should be limited. Omega-3 can also be found in walnuts, soybeans, beans, winter squash, avocados, and their seeds and oils. Only supplement Omega-3 if a nutritionist or physician has recommended you to do so.

Omega-6 fatty acids, also known as Lenoleic acid is important within food consumption but its effects are only positive if balanced with appropriate amounts of Omega-3. Too much Omega-6 encourages an inflammatory

> Did you know that farm raised fish contain more Omega-6 fatty acids than do wild caught fish?

response, increases the risk of coronary heart disease and other illnesses, and may counter the anti-inflammatory effects of Omega-3. Consuming too much Omega-6, may increasing your risk for cancer, particularly breast cancer in postmenopausal women (ExRx.net, 2014). Sounds pretty bad right? Well our body's aren't meant to host or consume large amounts of Omega-6 fatty acids as the fat within our bodies are mostly MUFAs and saturated fat. The imbalance of consuming too many Omega-6 fatty acids come when we eat products that have concentrated amounts of Omega-6 for the purpose of maintaining shelf life and taste. Consuming Omega-6 fatty acids in its natural form from plants, cereals, some nuts, whole grains, vegetable oils, meats, eggs, and milk, assist Omega-3 in providing positive changes within the body. In order to see the positive attributes of Omega-6 and Omega-3 fatty acids, it is recommended that you consume a 2:1 or 4:1 ratio. Unfortunately the average American has a 15:1 average consumption of Omega-6 to Omega-3 diet. Though this is partly due to standard farming techniques of grain feeding animals and production practices, we can do much better. Americans tend to not get enough Omega-3 fatty acids in their diet and are typically recommended to increase the foods that are abundant in this essential fat.

Trans-fat, typically listed on a nutrition label as "partially hydrogenated oil" is the result of a manufacturing process that causes unsaturated fats to be solid at room temperature (remember, MUFAs and PUFAs are liquid at room temperature – told ya), mimicking the structure of saturated fatty acids in order to extend shelf life. Partially hydrogenated oils and trans-fats are dangerous fats that increase your LDL cholesterol higher than saturated fats. Be mindful of your nutrition labels when purchasing processed and canned foods. Foods that can be high in trans-fats are chips, crackers, cakes, peanut butter and margarine; if you are going to purchase these items, make sure they indicate "trans-fat free" on the label.

> Did you know that grain fed animals contain more Omega-6 fatty acids than Omega-3 fatty acids when compared to animals who freely graze?

Saturated fatty acids are primarily found in meat products such as milk, cream, cheese, and butter, and are solid at room temperature. These fats are also found in palm and coconut oil, and in foods such as cakes, pastries, biscuits, pies and pretty much anything that is creamy, buttery or rich. Saturated fat is not an essential fat as it can be synthesized within the body, but it is very difficult to eradicate saturated fats from the diet and I personally do not suggest this. My goal is to teach you healthy habits that you can happily apply and maintain, not impossible suggestions that are only based upon science and not reality.

Many believe that if they decrease total fat intake as opposed decreasing total calorie intake, they have acquired the best opportunity for weight loss but this is incorrect. Solely focusing on reducing fat intake produces very little, if any, changes in body fat mass. The RDA for total fat intake is 20-35% of your diet, I recommend staying within the range of 20-25% of your diet coupled with a 25-30% protein intake. Concerning the breakdown of fat intake, > 7% of your fat intake should come from saturated fat, >1% from trans-fats, and roughly 15% PUFAs and 10% MUFAs.

Sample caloric intake percentages for optimal weight loss:

- 45% carbs, 30% protein, 25% fat
- 50% carbs, 30% protein, 20% fat
- 55% carbs, 25% protein, 20% fat

> *"Doing the best at this moment puts you in*
> *the best place for the next moment."*
> *–Oprah Winfrey*

The Impacts of Digestive Health on Weight Loss

Digestive System

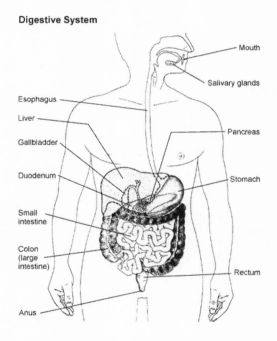

Digestion, and the health of the digestive system plays an important role in weight loss and maintaining a healthy lifestyle. Digestion is simply a system where the body breaks down the large food products you consumed, into small enough particles that can be absorbed into the blood stream and repurposed for energy. Digestion is the breakdown of your mashed potatoes, broccoli with cheese and chicken into carbs, fats and proteins allowing them to be reabsorbed into the body, and concluding with the excretion of waste.

Every carb is broken down into glucose and every protein is broken down into amino acids which are known as the building blocks of protein. Fat, on the other hand, is either broken down into free fatty acids, or triglycerides (three fatty acid molecules that are attached to a glycerol). You typically see triglycerides stored within muscle or liver while free fatty acids are found in the blood stream because fat is another source of energy.

Here's how digestion works: digestion begins in the mouth as saliva combined with chewing begins to soften, moisten and breakdown the forkful of food. After swallowing, this mass of food is now called a food bolus and muscles assist in moving the bolus through the esophagus into the stomach. Chemical fluids such as hydrochloric acid, bicarbonates and enzymes assist in the further decomposition of the bolus in the stomach. After the bolus combines with the stomach fluids, it is now called chyme which is the substance that leaves the stomach and enters the small intestine after being in the stomach for 2-4 hours. Also note that carbs are emptied first from the stomach into the intestines, followed by proteins and fats due to their chemical makeup. The majority of digestion occurs through the walls of the small intestine and food typically travels this 22-foot tube for 1-3 hours while further being diluted and broken down into absorbable molecules. As food is being broken down and the muscle actions of the small intestine pushes the chyme further along, it is the important role of indigestible fibers to clean the intestine and push along the residual chyme. After digestion has occurred, the small intestine then absorbs the nutrients and energy from chyme into the blood stream which shoots directly to the liver for processing and distribution of nutrients to the remainder of the body. The balance of chyme that is not absorbed gets pushed to the large intestine (colon) where the majority of water and some minerals are absorbed. Along with indigestible fiber, chyme is then released from the body as waste. As more water gets absorbed from the colon, the waste passing through it (the colon) begins to harden until its final excretion from the anus. If you have issues with hard stool, try drinking an extra glass of water and increasing your fiber intake, during and after your meal which will satisfy your large intestine's draw of water and it will soften your stool. The total time one meal can spend being digested from fork to waste is 18-72 hours therefore, a normal bowl movement frequency ranges from 3 times per day to once every 3 days, dependent on how frequently you eat. A simple way to track the heath of your gastrointestinal system is to track your bowl movements as they should follow the schedule of your eating habits.

The proper function of the digestive system positively effects weight loss. If your digestive system is sluggish and not functioning optimally, your body will not be able to utilize the foods that you've

> Did you know that caffeine causes triglycerides, which are stored fat, to breakdown into free fatty acids and enter the blood stream to be used as energy?

consumed nor will it be able to properly dispose of it. According to many experts, a weak digestive system can lead to fatigue, headaches, depression and inevitably weight gain. Without proper digestive functions, nutrients have a difficult time being absorbed for utilization within the body which is sometimes due to gunk blocking the absorptive pathways inside the small intestine. Without proper absorption, nutrients are not provided to the body's cells which are in need of energy, those cells then send signals to the brain and stomach begging for food because they are not receiving adequate nourishment. You may interpret these signals as hunger which drives you to eat more thus increasing total caloric intake without increasing the calories you burn, consequently leading to weight gain.

Here are ways to improve your digestive health and assist you in weight loss:

- **Eat less.** Many times we scarf down food without chewing adequately and not drinking sufficient amounts of water. With a large food bolus and little water, nutrients have less of an opportunity to be exposed to the walls of the small intestine for absorption. It is my suggestion to minimize the portion sizes you are currently eating to the size of your fist and to consume 5-6 meals per day. Increasing the number of times you eat will increase the amount of time your metabolism is active and burning calories while also decreasing the blood sugar peaks and valleys causing you metabolism to be active throughout the day.

- **Improve meal timing.** In order to consume 5-6 meals a day, I suggest eating 3 small meals, and 3 large snacks 3 hours in between. Refer back to Jessica's meal schedule for an example.

- **Eat more fiber.** As explained above, fiber acts as the push-broom of the intestines and it assists with the movement and clean-up of chyme and waste. As fiber pushes through your system, it cleans the small intestine increasing the surface area available for chyme to come in contact with the walls of the small intestine for absorption. Constipation, bloating, gas and hard stool are all consequences of a low fiber lifestyle.

Design Your Body Weekly Fitness Challenge: Eat Close to the Field

This Week's Challenge is to simply, eat close to the field by eating a salad a day. For some of you this may be the most difficult challenge yet!

Eating close to the field refers to eating fresher foods that contain the least amounts of processing possible.

Take a picture of the healthy foods you purchase from the market or foods that you eat and post it to my wall.

Good nutrition is a vital portion of your health and fitness goal. Eat at least 1 salad a day along with your exercise and watch your body change.

Daily Nutrition Log

Because of the importance of tracking what you eat, use the below food log to chart your daily food intake. Tracking what you eat drastically increases the chances that you will continue to eat healthy. Most people generally know what is and is not healthy and asking them to chart their habits will allow them to become more accountable and conscious towards the foods they eat. Carry this chart with you and at each meal, and jot down everything that you eat.

It is better to chart in the moment versus logging later in the day as it is easy to forget what you've eaten, bias can quickly set in, and life always tends to get in the way.

Make the time and make the commitment to yourself. This simple chart can be copied and reused daily. If you prefer technology over pen and paper, there are hundreds of nutrition journaling aps that you can look into, such as MyFitnessPal®, which are helpful tools to not only track what you are eating, but also gage your total calorie intake.

When using this chart, the rows indicate which meal or snack of the 3/3/3 you are charting, and the columns give detail about each meal or snack. For "Food/Beverage" you area to chart exactly what you ate/drank down to condiments and additives. The "Food Group & Serving" column asks you to chart what food group (s) are associated with your meal and the number of servings you consumed. In the next column, the goal is to chart how hungry you feel on a scale of one (not hungry at all) to five (extremely hungry). The column entitled, "Location & Emotion" is extremely important as this will help you chart and recognize patterns in your eating based upon intangible factors. Some people may eat differently based upon where they are and, in particular, what emotion they are experiencing at meal time and also if they are eating in response to emotion. The last column is a place for you to jot down other notes which may be helpful for your reference. Remember, each table is for 1 day. I suggest you copy this table, cut and paste it into each page of a new notebook that will become your nutrition journal as you begin to journal each day of your new lifestyle. For information on the up-to-date dietary guidelines visit www.health.gov/dietaryguidelines.

Coach Cailah's Food Log

Date:_____	Food/Beverage content	Food Group & Serving	Hunger Level (1-5)	Location & Emotion	Other Comments
Breakfast					
Snack					
Lunch					
Snack					
Dinner					
Snack					

For more information on gathering specific guidance in association with your age, height, weight, gender and activity level, visit www.choosemyplate.gov.

To clearly wrap up nutrition, here are a few guidelines to start your new lifestyle. Good nutrition or living healthy isn't about not eating, or only eating salad, it is about changing your thinking and controlling your desires. Sure, we all may want a cupcake, ice cream, cookies and whatever sweet treat tickles your fancy. But your temporary want should not dictate your actions. Don't let your impulses control your life. Control your own thoughts, decisions and actions. Having the impulse or desire to eat sweets or greasy food will not cease, but you will become stronger in making better decisions. It is acceptable to eat treats and "unhealthy" foods every-so-often, but limit those options to one cheat meal/week. If you have a high calorie day, your goal should be to balance those calories in with an extra hard workout to increase your calories out. When reviewing your nutrition log, begin to recognize your patterns and make adjustments accordingly. You may recognize that you eat more or particular foods depending on your mood or location. Once you've made this discovery, make a conscious decision to change it.

Throughout this chapter you've learned a lot of information on good nutrition and how to put it into practice, but I didn't directly tell you what to eat. My goal is to teach you how to fish, not to hand you the fish. But, since you invested in me, I'll invest in you. Here are a few tips and tricks to eating healthy:

- **Eat light.** Heavy meals are usually higher in calories. Eating light also reflects how you cook. If you decide to eat heavy, say you are at a family function or you go out to eat, choose items that have the best nutritional value. As opposed to a burger, grab steak and potatoes. Eating light doesn't mean you'll go hungry, you will still eat and be satisfied, but the goal is to decrease the amount of calories it takes for you to be satisfied.
- **Only eat until satisfied.** Americans overeat. We overeat because the food tastes good and simply because we can. If you are eating until you physically cannot stuff anything else in your mouth, than you have far surpassed your limit. At the end of each meal

you should not have to unbutton your pants or sit back to give your belly room to expand. Eat until you are satisfied, or no longer hungry, even if there is food still left on your plate. Don't worry, I'm not encouraging you to waste food. When you have reached the point where you are satisfied, save the rest of your meal for your next snack. Point blank; don't overeat.

- **Eat often.** Keep your metabolism as steady as possible by eating 5-6 meals per day. Your goal is to stick to my 3-3-3 rule: 3 small meals, 3 large snacks, 3 hours in between each. Do not skip meals.

- **Create a routine.** If you exercise Mondays, Wednesdays and Fridays, add more protein throughout those days. Have eggs for breakfast as opposed to a smoothie or cereal. On the days where you don't exercise, it is acceptable to have lower caloric intake due to the decrease in activity requirements. Put your body on a schedule of when to eat and what types of food you should eat.

- **Meal prep.** Take time the night before, or a few days out to plan your meals. Plan your meals before grocery shopping, and only shop for the week. Plan to "eat close to the ground" and challenge yourself to have as many colors in each meal as possible.

- **Be careful with carbs.** Note the differences between simple and complex carbs and how they affect your body. Typically our diets are grain and protein rich whereas if we exchanged more fruits and veggies for some carbs and proteins, we would decrease the total amount of carbs we ingest, therefore decreasing the potential for weight gain.

- **Eat simple.** I was raised to eat richly, and like most African American families in the United States, the majority of my elders have high blood pressure and diabetes. We love to cook and we love to eat. Though I am living healthier than how I was raised, I still love to cook and eat! I have learned to exchange fat and oil as flavor substitutes for seasonings and the natural flavor of foods and the millions of combinations they bring.

- **Explore your grocery store.** There are many foods with health benefits that you do not eat as it hasn't been passed down to you. Example, I never heard of couscous until I entered graduate school and studied nutrition more closely, and there were many foods like mangos, tuna and even barley that I've heard of but never tried on my own. This was never a staple in my family dishes but now I have branched out and have expanded my refrigerator and therefore ability to cook more flavorful foods. Enjoy this process and create an experiment in your kitchen.
- **Eat before you workout.** Research suggests that people who eat (typically simple carbs before the workout) lose more weight than those who do not incorporate a pre-workout meal.

"Let thy food be thy medicine and thy medicine be thy food."
-Hippocrates

CHAPTER 6

General Exercise

Millions of individuals are attempting to control and lose weight. Based on a study done in 2000, 46% of women and 33% of men reported their attempts at weight loss but most did not incorporate an increased level of physical activity or exercise, therefore they did not reach their initial goals (ACE - American Council on Exercise, 2011, p. 201).

Many nutritionists over amplify the importance of nutrition, saying that weight loss is 90% contingent upon what you eat. I disagree. Nutrition is an important aspect of weight loss along with exercise. Without exercise, reaching your weight loss goals become more and more difficult as you can only limit your caloric intake to a specific point before it becomes unhealthy and your body enters a catabolic state. If I were to place a numerical figure on the importance of nutrition and exercise I would landmark them as having an equally important relationship of 50:50. With the absence of adequate exercise there is a floor to weight loss that many people encounter which would otherwise be an easy breakthrough. The same is true with exercise only.

"Don't you know that your body is a temple of the Holy Spirit which is in you, which has been given to you from God?... For you were bought with a price: glorify God therefore in your body."
-1 Corinthians 6:19-20

What You Should Know Before Engaging in Exercise:

- Rapid weight loss can be dangerous and cause serious health problems. In order to deter unnecessary health complications it is advised to remain within the range of 1-2lbs of weight loss per week, or less than 1% of body weight lost in a two week period.
- Only *permanent* lifestyle changes such as improved nutrition (increasing vegetables, fruits and lean protein intake) and increased physical activity (exercise, walking, playing, weightlifting etc.) promote long-term weight loss.
- Complete your PAR-Q in Chapter 1 and consult your physician as needed.
- If you are engaging a personal trainer, health coach or another exercise professional, request their qualifications to make sure they are certified and legitimized.

Preparing for Exercise

Now that we've become more active by following the baby steps of increasing activity in Chapter 2, we are now able to get a little more serious. Always remember that exercise has the potential to be hazardous to your health as it can cause injury and potentially death if not followed correctly. Progression is key. Do not jump into marathon running, sprinting, high intensity training or various exercise that you are unfamiliar with or that you haven't performed in some time. Again, progression is the key to a healthy and safe exercise session along with increasing the possibility of you sticking with the program you've created.

One of your time sensitive goals should be to drop 10% of your body weight in six months' time. This is done by steadily increasing your activity and beginning from the basics, even if you were a former athlete. Beginning an exercise program is just like getting into a pool. Some may dive in without even looking to see how deep or shallow the pool is. If you have not exercised in more than four months, I strongly encourage you to put your toes in, followed by your calves, then thighs, waist, chest, then full body; just start slow.

At every exercise session you should bring a bottle of water, a towel, your music (if you prefer) and an accountability partner on deck. Water is often overlooked as not being an important component of good health when truthfully, it is as important as oxygen. The loss of total body water can cause dangerous and counter effective results in the body such as decreased blood volume, impaired physical performance, nausea, difficulty concentrating, dizziness, weakness, muscle spasms, delirium and death if the total body water lost is greater than 20%. Outside of being the single largest component in your body, water has an innumerable amount of positive effects and necessities for the body; drink more water.

Note there are five components of physical fitness: cardiovascular endurance, muscle endurance, muscle strength, flexibility and body composition. This book focuses on improving each component as each have the ability to drastically impact your health and weight loss. Each of your exercise sessions should focus on at least three of the five. The two I am making mandatory for each session is flexibility and body composition. You may then choose your third focus of either one or a combination of the following; cardiovascular endurance, muscle strength or muscle endurance for each session. Exercises that work towards improving neuromuscular fitness such as stability, balance and agility should also be incorporated, particularly for older adults, and those with joint issues or instabilities.

In order to be successful, set your mind on positivity and nonstop action, cut off all other options and DECIDE to be successful.

Popup Coach: Now that we've finally gotten to exercise instruction, challenge yourself to read and act on everything you learn in this book. Put yourself on a regimen, and put yourself on the track for success and weight loss. View and take part in this "30 Day Fitness Challenge" video. Though it says for summer, don't worry about the dates, challenge yourself and jump start your system with this Design Your Body Fitness Challenge. https://www.youtube.com/watch?v=4efUfQD0IOA

Warm Up, Cool Down and Flexibility

It's time to get started!! Anytime you exercise you want to prepare your body for the stress you are about to put it through. Your warm up should include all major muscle groups with a focus on the muscles you will exercise during that session, whether your workout consists of cardio or resistance training. Engaging in at least a 5-10 minute full body warm up will increase body temperature, heart rate, blood flow, joint lubrication, muscle and tissue elasticity and your body's ability to respond to different stimuli. Participating in warm up will make it harder for you to sustain a musculoskeletal injury. Flexibility is also an extremely important part of the warm up. Stretching further prepares your muscles and joints for the stress ahead and it also decreases injury potential to muscle tissue.

Increasing your flexibility is important for muscle function and potentially muscle growth. When static stretching, spend at least 20 seconds on each muscle group. Include large muscles such as chest and glutes, along with small muscles like calves or the muscles in your forearm. To ensure you are hitting every muscle group, start from the top and work your way down.

My stretching order:

- **Breathing and upper body:** Lace your fingers together and each up and touch the sky. Lean to your right and hold for 20s, lean to your left and hold for 20s.
- **Arm Circles:** 10 large arm circles front, and 10 large arm circles back.
- **Shoulders:** Right arm crosses in front of your chest and over the left arm, take your left hand and grab your right elbow and pull to your chest. Reverse.
- **Triceps:** Raise your right arm above your head with your palm facing behind you, bend at the elbow until your palm touches

your upper back, take your left hand, grab your elbow and pull down. Reverse.

- **Biceps/forearms:** Stretch your right arm in front of you with your palm facing up, take your left hand and grab your right palm and pull your right hand back toward your elbow.
- **Core:** Standing with your feet shoulder width apart, and a slight bend, twist side to side 20 times total.
- **Hamstrings:** With your legs straight but not locked out, bend over and touch your toes. Reach as far as you can and grab you knees, calves, and ankles or touch the floor depending on your level of flexibility.
- **Quadriceps:** While still standing, balance on your left leg (it is OK to hold on to something if you need to) bend your right knee and bring your right heel close to your butt. Grab your right foot with your right hand and lightly pull. Reverse.
- **Upper Leg:** Standing with your legs wide, lunge to the right allowing your left toe to point towards the ceiling while your left heel is on the ground. In lunging to the right with this stretch you may balance on the ball of your foot while allowing your right glute to get as close as it can to your right heel. Place your hands flat on the ground, your left hand on the left side of your right foot, and the right hand on the right side of your foot. After 20s of lunging, slowly straighten your right leg by pushing upward and keeping your hands on the ground and hold for 20 or more seconds. Keep your hands on the ground and walk them over to your left leg and repeat.
- **Inner Thigh:** Spread your legs as wide as you can, bend over and place both hands on the floor and stretch. You may grab both ankles if you see fit. After 20 or more seconds, walk your feet together in preparation for the next stretch.
- **Calves:** Walk to a wall and place the ball of your right foot on the wall while your right heel stays on the ground. Lean towards the

wall and stretch. This may also be done by standing on stairs and allowing your heels to sink below the ledge of the step.

Just as the warm up prepares your body for exercise, the cool down is just as important as transitioning from a state of exercise to a state of homeostasis. The cool down is purposed to slowly bring your body's core temperature and heart rate closer to resting levels. There are dangers associated with going from a state of exercise to immediately resting. Without getting into the extreme physiological science of this matter, it is better to progress your body into a slower heart rate as this is more advantageous for good heart health and safety.

Cool downs also protect against Delayed Onset Muscle Soreness (DOMS) which occurs as a result of heavy muscle use and soreness sets in 24-48 hours after the exercise session. Stretching and slow cardio assists with transporting chemicals such as hydrogen ions, the thing that makes you "feel the burn", and inflammation away from the muscle, therefore, decreasing future soreness. As you exercise, blood flow is redirected from organs to active muscles and other tissues to provide more oxygen and fuel for action. One of the many jobs of muscles is to assist with pushing blood back to the heart to be refueled and redistributed. If you immediately sit down after exercise, this muscle pumping action discontinues and less blood is returned to the heart and therefore the brain causing dizziness (due to lack of oxygen) and potentially nausea. Progressively slowing the action of your muscles by participating in low intensity cardio and stretching deters this from occurring as the muscle pump has not stopped pushing blood back to the heart for redistribution.

Your typical exercise session (ACSM, 2010, p. 154):

- 10 min walk/jog or other light cardio (40-60% max effort) and 10 min stretch or dynamic stretch for warm up →
- 20-60min conditioning of cardio, resistance, neuromuscular and/or sports related activities (40-80% max effort). Exercise

bouts of 10 mins are adequate as long as you accumulate at least 20 mins. →

- 10 min walk/jog or other light cardio (60-40% max effort) for cool down.

Incorporating a warm up and cool down into each exercise session will ensure creating the environment for the safest and most effective weight loss to take place.

General Exercise Recommendations for Healthy Adults

Weekly Frequency in days/week (d/wk)	Do These Types of Exercises
At least 5d/wk	Moderate intensity (40-60% max effort) activities of aerobic, weight bearing and flexibility exercises.
At least 3d/wk	Vigorous intensity ($\geq$ 60% max effort) aerobic, weight bearing and flexibility activities.
3-5d/wk	A combination of moderate and vigorous intensity aerobic activities, weight-bearing exercise and flexibility exercise.
2-3d/wk	Muscular strength and endurance, resistance exercises, calisthenics, balance and agility

(ACSM, 2010, p. 153)

"If you want the body of an athlete, you have to train like one"
-Cailah Brock

Steps to Writing Your Exercise Plan – FITT Principles

The FITT Principals are the bricks and mortar to creating your exercise plan. This is how you detail your workouts and create a progressive plan that pushes you closer to your destination. Remember, this journey never truly ends, once you reach a level of satisfaction with your health, you must still maintain that lifestyle. The acronym FITT stands for Frequency, Intensity, Time and Type. Combining these four areas will create a seamless exercise plan for you to follow and are the principles on which to base your exercise. After reading the FITT principles, look at the example exercise Plan for tips on creating your own.

* The below suggestions are not for women who are pregnant

Frequency

Frequency is defined as the number of days per week that are dedicated to an exercise program via physical activity or exercise. The U.S. Surgeon General and other U.S. government agencies recommend participating in exercise and/or physical activity on all or most days of the week. Yup, that is a 5-7 day workout routine. The majority of Americans do not meet these standards, by creating a progressive exercise plan, you and I will slowly reach our way to meeting this exercise expectation. The American College of Sports Medicine (ACSM) has also found that the benefits of exercise can be seen with 3-5d/wk of both moderate and vigorous exercise provide substantial results and if nothing else, we will set our first goals for meeting this criteria.

Moderate aerobic activity can be performed 5d/wk while vigorous aerobic or resistance training is best when performed 3d/wk. My suggestion is combining and alternating days of moderate and vigorous activity on a weekly schedule of 3-5d/wk in order to achieve and maintain health and fitness benefits.

Intensity

Exercise intensity denotes how hard your body is working during a bout of exercise. According to the ACSM, "There is a positive continuum of health/fitness benefits with increasing exercise intensity." (ACSM, 2010, p. 155). Plainly stated, the harder you work, the better and faster health benefits you will see. Reversely, a minimum threshold exists for gaining benefits from physical activity and exercise and many individuals are "exercising" below this threshold and are not seeing the results they desire.

There is a difference between physical activity and exercise. Physical activity is activity that requires your body to move at a higher intensity than at resting homeostasis, but not intense enough to be categorized as exercise. Some examples of physical activity are; cleaning, cooking, grocery shopping, playing, laughing, crying, short bouts of walking, stairs, and anything that increases your heart rate, breathing and core temperature, but not enough to cause sweating. The onset of sweating typically occurs while exercising at 40-60% of maximal effort and is the minimal recommendation for adults to achieve health and fitness benefits. The best health and fitness related results are seen with combining moderate and vigorous exercises ≥60% maximal effort. With this said, you have to be willing to push yourself out of your comfort zone in order to see the results you want. One tough workout isn't enough for results, your exercise needs to continually go beyond your comfort zone for best results. Still listen to your body with injuries, heart palpitations etc., but push yourself towards success.

In order to tell how hard you are working during exercise, and a great way to plan the intensity/vigorousness of your exercises is to base intensity on your heart rate. Your intensity will be based on your predicted heart rate max (HRmax) which has a familiar calculation of 220-age. Though widely used for its ease, it is variable in its accuracy. This formula underestimates both male and female HRmax for those < 40 while overestimating HRmax for both sexes > 40 which is extremely dangerous. The more accurate representation of your HRmax that I use in calculating my client's target exercise zones is:

$$HRmax = 206.9 - (0.67 \text{ X age})$$

List your HRmax: _____

Now that you have found the indicator of your maximal effort, you are better able to track your body's response to exercise. For example, if your HRmax is 178bpm and your intensity goal in a particular exercise session is 68%, your target HR should be 121bpm. Basing exercise intensity on your age-predicted HRmax is beneficial for all except those who take beta-blockers as they affect how the heart responds to activity. It is to your benefit to invest in a HR monitor.

The Rate of Perceived Exertion (RPE) is also an effective scale of dictating exercise intensity. The RPE is a scale that is typically used 6-20 but for the sake of simplicity you may use the modified scale 1-10; 1 being lying in bed on a lazy Saturday morning and 10 being all out maximal effort running from lions, tigers and bears. In using the 1-10 RPE scale, your goal for moderate intensity days are scores of 5-6, and your goal for vigorous days are scores of 7-9. Varying the level of intensity per exercise day will give you a drastic boost in your exercise and health benefits.

Your exercise intensity should be varied on a day-to-day basis. Combinations of moderate (40-60% HRmax) and vigorous (60-80% HRmax) exercise have been proven to provide the most beneficial health and fitness responses in most adults. This is extremely important when creating your exercise plan. If you use all the tips I provide, you will steadily achieve success. The lack of intensity is one of the main reasons people do not lose the weight they wish. Below is an example of a 4d/wk exercise intensity schedule. Whether you exercise 4 days or 2 days, create and chart your intensity and off days so you can truly Design Your Body.

Sample Intensity Schedule

Monday	80% HRmax or 7-8 RPE
Tuesday	60% HRmax or 5-6 RPE
Wednesday	OFF
Thursday	80% HRmax or 7-8 RPE
Friday	OFF
Saturday	60% HRmax or 5-6 RPE
Sunday	OFF

Design Your Body Weekly Fitness Challenge: 1 Mile Run for Time

Whether you run mileage throughout the week or you complain about a busy schedule, this challenge is for you. Get away from your mundane schedule and check this out.

My Current Walkers: Amp up the intensity of your workout and try and get one mile as fast as you can. This means step up your speed and start jogging. Each time you try the challenge, you should shoot for a faster time.

My current runners: As opposed to just running for distance, switch up your program and run a short distance for time, as fast as you can. This means no jogging, no puttering, and crank up the intensity! Varying your workouts is an awesome way to get better and faster results. Sometimes, long is wrong.

My "I have no free time" peoples: Most people can hit one mile in less than 25 minutes. That's it! Get up, set aside 25 minutes of your time and start moving. Stop putting off your weight loss and get up to get to it!

I CHALLENGE YOU to post your one mile time on my wall. Don't worry about other people's times, your journey is your own and be proud of your progress. Every time you run a mile this week, post your time on my wall so we can keep track of your progress. Try this challenge at least 3 times (3 miles in 7 days NOT DIFFICULT!). Changing up your workout will help you burn more fat and more total calories (Y).

Switch it up with this Challenge!

Time

Exercise quantity and duration are both references to the amount of time spent exercising. Since exercise frequency is how many d/wk you are exercising, time is total workout duration per training session. Your goal should be 60mins of activity in each exercise session. Due to the dose-response relationship between exercise and calories burned/week, the absolute minimum amount of exercise you should get is 30mins on all or most days of the week. If your schedule only permits for 30mins of training, increase you training intensity for that section by either going faster or harder or even adding interval training. This will increase total calories burned and maintain training quality. The purpose of endurance is to determine how long your cardiovascular system or muscular system can sustain a particular activity. The stronger these systems, the more generally healthy you are.

The U.S. Surgeon General, ACSM and the American Heart Association (AHA) recommend at least 1,000cal burned via physical activity per week. One thousand calories are equivalent to roughly 150mins of exercise/wk or 30min/d of exercise. For individuals trying to lose weight, the above organizations and I, recommend a larger quantity of calories burned which will result in greater health and fitness benefits. Set your exercise goal to burn around 2,000cals/week which equates to 200-300min/wk or 30-50min/d. Currently, there is no maximal volume of exercise (unlike food where there is a maximum and minimum you should intake). As your program progresses you may wish to begin competing in sports, running or fitness competitions, possibly dictating which a higher range of calories burned/wk, but otherwise your program should be based on 250-300mins/week of activity.

Exercises performed for at least 30mins/d on more than 5d/wk for a total of 150 or more minutes is suggested for moderate intensity activity. Engaging in vigorous activity should be done 3-5d/wk for 20-25mins/ session for a total of 75mins/wk. In order to participate in an effective weight loss program, shoot for 300mins of moderate activity or 150mins of vigorous activity or a combination of the two for 3-5d/wk (ACSM, 2010, p. 163). In beginning your exercise plan, it may be appropriate to begin with 3-5 bouts of 10min exercises on all or most days of the week which still provides some positive health benefits albeit much slower than my recommendations above.

Type

When you exercise, you should do it for a purpose, bka train. Training for weight loss should incorporate many different types of exercise such as training for agility, speed, cardiovascular endurance, muscle strength, flexibility, power and muscle endurance. Though you may not think it, each type of training is necessary for you to maintain a healthy progression during your weight loss journey as well as deter injuries and other problems that result from the physiological changes of adapting to a smaller body. Each of these exercise types fall under cardiovascular or resistance training. Endurance activities typically require minimal skill or effort due to their repetitive nature. Developing muscle strength is accomplished by fighting against resistance, whether an external weight or gravity (body weight exercises). Training for balance is often not on people's agenda but it has great potential to decrease injuries from falls, and the occurrence of muscle tares as balance is simply training your neuromuscular system to fire faster and more effectively. Agility training refers to the ability and effectiveness of changing direction quickly which is a requirement for multidirectional athletes (such as basketball, volleyball, football, soccer etc.) along with being extremely helpful in generating quick movements that are needed (catching a cup that falls from the shelf). Training for power is extremely important for all populations. Since power = force X velocity, power is a relationship of force (the ability to generate strength) and speed (or agility/quickness). To put this in more practical terms: if you slip while exiting the shower and are able to act quickly enough to grab the shower rail and exert enough force on that rail to counter the force of your body falling, you have demonstrated adequate amounts of power to stop yourself from falling. This is extremely important in the elderly population, particularly as they age because bone density decreases while increasing brittleness, especially if they are not engaged in a resistance training program.

I'd like to introduce you to a few of my favorite styles of exercise that you should incorporate into your training regimen.

- **Interval Training:** Interval training is simply alternating work and rest periods of exercise. Example; run 45s, walk 15s repetitively for 30mins. Interval training burns high amounts of calories and is my best recommendation for you. Interval training burns more calories than Long Slow Distance (LSD). This is due to the energy it takes for your body to a.) complete the exercise b.) slow itself down to near resting levels from exercise during your rest period, and c.) increase body activity to exercise again. Add the energy requires to slow yourself down then bring your body back to a state of exercise, multiplied by the number of times you are doing that set of activities. Long Slow Distance training only burns calories during one exercise and one rest session. Interval training has the potential to double and triple the effects and calorie burn found in LSD. This concept is referred to as Excess Post-exercise Oxygen Consumption.
- **High Intensity Interval Training (HIIT):** The same as interval training but its focus is on alternating between high intensity activities, whereas interval training can be variations of low or moderate intensity exercises. Example; 60s pull ups, 60s push-ups, 60s plank, 2min rest 7 times total. This style of training burns the most calories, though it cannot be maintained for long periods of time. Be careful if you decide to engage in this style of exercise training, and make sure you are properly progressing by increasing exercise duration first, then intensity, then changing exercise type. Without proper progression into HIIT, you are at an increased risk of musculoskeletal and cardiovascular injury.

- **Long Slow Distance (LSD):** LSD training is my least favorite, this is participating in cardiovascular exercises such as running, for long periods of time (<60mins). This type of exercise can be completed on a moderate intensity day as high intensities cannot be achieved with LSD. However, long durations can be accomplished.

- **Weight Bearing vs Non-Weight Bearing Activities:** Regardless of cardio or resistance training, a combination of weight baring and non-weight baring activities are important to your health. Referring to the SAID principle, your bones adapt to the stresses placed upon them just like any other tissue in your body (assuming the stress isn't overwhelming). When we walk, run, jump, change direction and lift weights, our bones are forced to grow and adapt in order to maintain proper support of the activities we engage in. As we age, our bone mineral density deteriorates causing bones to become more fragile and brittle due to reduced activity. In order to stop this natural process of deterioration due to underuse, you must increase the stress on your skeletal system in order for your bones to grow and adapt. Non-weight baring activities such as swimming, elliptical, recumbent bike, and arm bikes are also positive to engage in on lower intensity days. Just as your tissue needs rest and repair time, your bones do as well. Weight baring activities, along with adequate calcium intake assist in the improvement of bone health.

In conjunction with the FITT principles of exercise, there is a fifth principle that isn't commonly added, but it is one whose omission is the main reason why health seekers plateau during exercise. Without the insertion of a proper *progression* plan for frequency, intensity, time, and type, health seekers have a much more difficult time in progressing towards success. As stated above, the SAID principle (Specific Adaptations for Imposed Demand) dictates that your body will adapt to the stresses placed upon it. Engaging in the same routine allows your body to adapt to that stressor and eventually your body gets to the point where it isn't as challenged as it once was. As your body reaches this point, less energy is required to perform the same functions (because your body has become more efficient and completing the same task), therefore less calories are burned and those seeking weight loss may not find it once their progress has plateaued. Plateaus are simply the point where your body has adapted to a particular stressor at a near maximal level and it is in need of a different type of stress or exercise.

Time is the first principle of FITT you should progress in your cardiovascular endurance program. An increase in exercise time of 5-10mins (5-10lbs for resistance training) every 1-2 weeks is an adequate progression for the first 4-6 weeks of activity. After you have been consistently exercising for over a month, frequency and intensity are the next principles to increase in both your cardio and resistance training programs. Exercise frequency can be increased by increasing the number of days you do that particular exercise, or increasing the total number of days you exercise in general. Exercise intensity is increased by increasing how hard you work as quantified by HRmax and RPE (remember your calculations and Rate of Perceived Exertion scale from above). Varying your exercises also increases exercise intensity. Example, while keeping frequency and time the same, exercise intensity can be accomplished by changing from interval training to LSD, or by increasing the speed of your walk/jog, or even adding hills to your exercise. Intensity is also increased by stepping up how hard the exercise is for you. Gradually increase your exercise intensity and frequency for the next 4-6 months. After 6 months of varying your frequency, intensity, time and type, it is time to completely change your exercise routine by revamping your entire program with new exercise, new cardio and adding accountability partners to exercise with you.

There are the progressions to each FITT principle which should be used in order. This is the key to creating your own exercise plan.

Sample Exercise Log:

Exercise	Frequency & Day of Week	Intensity	Time	Type	Progression
Cardio	3d/wk, MWF	60-80% Hrmax	45mins	Interval aTraining	Increase 5min/week
Resistance Training	2d/wk, TTH	50-60%Hrmax	1hr	3sets of 12 reps on machines	Start using dumbbells in week 4
Rest	2d/wk, SS	NA	NA	NA	NA

You can include in detail specific exercises such as walking, jogging, elliptical, swimming or biking in the Exercise Category, whose frequency can range from 1-7 days depending on how in love you are with that particular exercise. As long as you have 5 days of cardio and 2 days of resistance (you may do both cardio and resistance in the same day if you wish), Coach Cailah is happy. Plotting each exercise allows you to plan your week of training with the activities that will keep your interest. It also allows you to vary your intensities per exercise. Example, you may have a water aerobics class that you enjoy which can increase your HR to 78% HRmax on Tuesdays and Thursdays, while you spend your low intensity days on Wednesdays with exercising on the recumbent bike shooting for a 60% HRmax intensity. This is how exercise professionals plan their clients' exercise routines. The same holds true for resistance training. You should have a separate spreadsheet or logging section for your resistance exercises such as squats, leg press, bench press, biceps curls, triceps extension, shoulder press, calf raise, abdominal crunch, lat pulldown etc. This log should incorporate all the exercises you do in the gym as well as those you do at home. Here you can begin to create your exercise plan as you pick and choose what exercises to do on which days depending on your schedule of gym, home or outside (an Exercise Matrix is provided for you in Chapter 8). It is important to plot the intensity of each exercise (cardio and resistance) and more so, to plan the progression of each.

> **Design Your Body Weekly Fitness Challenges:**
>
> YOUR WEEKLY CHALLENGE:
> I challenge you to get 100+ abs per day, 100+ squats per day and 30+ pushups per day. This equals to 700 abs, 700 squats, and 210 pushups this week!
> You think it's too much? Try breaking it down like this:
> 20 abs 5x/day,
> 20 squats 5x/day and
> 5 pushups 6x/day.
>
> Being in shape is a total body experience. Many people want the abs, the firm butt and toned arms, but if you are not maintaining full body exercises, you won't reach or maintain the body you want.
> Yes indeed my friends summer is coming to an end so let's hit the next season running.
> No matter the struggle, no matter the journey, you have to opportunity to make your goals your personal duty.

Your Exercise Log:

Exercise	Frequency & Day of week	Intensity	Time	Type

Note: All exercise progressions should be done gradually and you should follow the guidelines above for progressing Time first, then Frequency, then Intensity and finally Type. Avoid large jumps in your progression plan to minimize the risk of muscle soreness and injury.

Note: Listen to your body when creating and following this plan. Muscle soreness will occur but there is a difference between muscle soreness and micro injuries. Keep water with you at all times when exercising, be cognizant of outdoor and indoor temperatures, and understand how your body responds to exercise. This book is a guide to creating an exercise plan for weight loss but you must take into consideration your own body and what works for you. As always, consult your physician with any questions you may have, and chart your body's responses to exercise. Just as you keep a nutrition log, keep an exercise log where you note the things your body is experiencing before and after exercise. Having this log will allow you to track patterns in your body which can indicate positive and negative side-effects of exercise. Heart palpitations, dizziness, unnatural shortness of break should be logged and reported to a physician. I encourage you to purchase a heart rate monitor which will assist you in tracking your intensity via HRmax percentages, but it can also track drastic fluctuations in your heart rate. If you are extremely overweight, you must take care in slowly progressing yourself into exercise as to decrease the risk of a cardiovascular event. The goal is to reduce injury and maximize results so take it slow and make your results last a lifetime.

CHAPTER 7

Cardiovascular Training

To begin, there are two ways to train your cardiovascular system; endurance training and interval or speed training. Both styles of training benefit the cardiovascular system by improving blood flow, blood volume, oxygen uptake, capillary density, heart health, hormone profiles and diabetic management just to name a few. Endurance training consists of any type of aerobic conditioning that is long in duration, has a rhythmic nature and utilizes large muscle groups. Examples of training for cardiovascular endurance are jogging, running, biking, elliptical, swimming, and skiing for long periods of time while focusing on increasing speed and distance. When training for 10Ks and other races, LSD is the best type of training to accomplish this goal. Training for speed and power is also an excellent consideration when creating your exercise plan.

Though you may not feel you should train like a track and field athlete, the benefits of interval training in the form of short quick runs or various bouts of cardio introduce a great advantage to weight loss as this style of training provides a higher level of calorie burn than does training LSD.

As stated above, interval training is my favorite style of training because you can get the same, if not better workout than you can with LSD in less time by raising your intensity. If you ranked your Cardio in the "poor" category based on the Trinity Figures Scale, LSD is your starting point. Here are a few exercise options and examples for LSD:

- 60 minute walk on treadmill or around the neighborhood
- 30minute swim
- 30minute jog
- 2mile jog
- 45mins on any piece of cardio equipment in the gym

There are two different ways to effectively train to improve your cardiovascular system while participating in LSD no matter what level you begin with. When participating in LSD, set your goals based on time or distance (notice how the above examples are a mixture of the two styles). When training for time, utilize anything with a known distance such as a track, a loop around the neighborhood or set a distance on the treadmill. Train yourself to complete that route faster than the previous attempt by increasing the speed/pace at which you walk/run. Complete the route with a moderate –fast pace, mark your time down and let this time be your baseline. Each time you attempt this route, you should complete it faster than the last.

These are examples of running a set distance with the focus of decreasing your time. The reverse focus is also a great benefit to weight loss. Select a time and shoot to cover the longest distance possible within the given timeframe. Example, imagine you only have 45minutes to workout, allow 15mins for your warm up and cool down and 30mins to complete your cardiovascular exercise. Your goal is to cover the maximal amount of distance possible within this time. This type of exercise works best on set loops, tracks and various cardiovascular equipment where you can quantify your results.

As your speed increases and exercise time decreases, you will flow away from the realm of LSD and you are prepared to begin interval training by increasing the repetitions of that particular exercise. Example, initially, you walk 2 miles on the treadmill which takes you 32 minutes to complete. Your set distance is 2 miles and each time you engage in this exercise, your goal is to get faster and faster. Eventually you reach the point where you run 2 miles in 20 minutes and you feel as if you can still do more. Here is the point where you should add another set or increase the distance. After your first set of 2mile jogging, rest for about 5-6 minutes, then begin your second set of 2 mile running (This is the beginning of interval training). Or run 3 miles for time.

Interval training is simply interchanging periods of work and rest. This has huge benefits to your system based on the science of EPOC. Your rest interval can range from seconds to minutes, just as your work intervals. Interval training can be completed with anything from cardio equipment to an open field and can be purposed for both cardio and resistance training. Here are a few examples of interval training for cardio:

- **Fartlek:** Known as "speed play" in German. When participating in this type of interval training you are sprinting/going as fast as you can for a certain period of time, followed by an equal period of active rest such as walking or jogging. This can resemble sprinting for 30s and jogging for 30s or running for 3mins and walking for 3mins for a particular distance or time.
- **Kenyan Runs:** This exercise idea came from one of my college coaches, and is a style of interval training that has set work and rest intervals. Kenyan run workout: 15s hard, 15s off, 30s hard, 30s off, 45s hard, 45s off and 60s hard, 60s off. Kenyan runs are repeated for total time or sets.

Personally, I hate running. Yup, I said it. I absolutely hate running. But I am fully aware of the extreme benefits associated with this painful act. I know a few friends in running clubs and these women run 15 or more miles a week but wonder why they aren't seeing the results they wish. In terms of cardiovascular fitness they are in decent shape, but the style of training

> **Design Your Body Fitness Challenge**
>
> 45 minute Interval training challenge. Run 2mins, walk/jog 1min until you reach 45mins for 3 workouts this week.

they are engaged in does not truly impact weight loss long term because they are only participating in one form of activity. When I train for a photo shoot, outside of dieting and cutting overall calories, I participate in interval training with both cardio and weights. For a typical training session in preparation for a photo shoot I will warm up, run one mile as fast as I can or interval train for 20mins, spend 1.5-2hrs lifting weights, then back to 30-50mins of LSD on the treadmill, elliptical or Stairmaster, or spend 10mins on each machine which combined gives me high level of calorie burn 5-6d/wk. Disclaimer: this is my high intensity workout and 24 years of consistent exercise allows my body to handle this extreme regimen and I do not recommend this to you. Notice I used the word "diet" which refers to a temporary state of nutrition and I'll include the temporary state of high intensity exercise. You are training to improve your life, not only training for one moment or occasion in your life. Use the guidelines set forth in this book to create an exercise plan tailored to fit you and you may eventually reach the point where you can safely complete the above exercises and I might just fly out to run you through a personal training with me. Imagine that!

When beginning your weight loss journey via cardiovascular fitness, I recommend beginning with LSD training. This will gradually progress your fitness level by increasing stamina, improving baseline cardiovascular fitness and by safely take off the weight that is easiest to rid yourself of. If you are new to exercise or you haven't exercised in the past 3 or more months, I recommend beginning with low intensity LSD training for 20-40 minutes 3-5d/wk for 3 weeks straight at 57-67% HRmax. If you ranked in the Poor or Average category of the Trinity Figures Scale, I recommend the above starting point. Yes, depending on your baseline fitness levels, you may need to start off slower than what you expected, but remember, this is a new lifestyle that you are creating. Just putting your toe in the pool may not be the cannon ball you expected, but it is the beginning of the lifelong swim you've been looking for. It'll work, trust me, and follow the guidelines to creating your plan.

As a refresher, your weight loss goal should be 1-2lbs/wk which relates to 3,500-7,000cals burned by a combination of diet and exercise, 10% of total weight lost by month 6, and a total exercise time of 200-300mins/wk with a combination of weight baring and non-weight baring activities.

Below is the framework set forth by the U.S. Department of Health and Human Services as recommendations for physical activity. This is the best option to choose your frequency, intensity and time/duration of exercise based on your current level of physical activity. Honestly assess yourself and refer back to the Trinity Figures Scale for Cardiovascular activity and use your results to pinpoint your exercise starting point.

Physical Activity Level	Fitness Classification	Frequency		Intensity		Time	
		Cals/wk	Days/wk	%Hrmax	Effort Put in Exercise	Duration/day	Duration/wk
Sedentary, no consistent exercise	Poor	500-1000	3-5d/wk	57-67%	Light-moderate	20-30mins	60-150mins
Little physical activity and very deconditioned	Poor-fair	1000-1500	3-5d/wk	64-74%	Light-moderate	30-60	150-200mins
Inconsistent physical activity, moderately to mildly deconditioned	Fair-average	1500-2000	3-5d/wk	74-54%	Moderate-hard	30-90mins	200-300mins
Consistently physically active and maintains exercise sessions that are moderate to vigorous intensity. (In shape)	Average-good	>2000	3-5d/wk	80-91%	Moderate-hard	30-90mins	200-300mins
High and consistent physical activity. Typical athletes	>Good-excellent	>2000	3-5d/wk	84-94%	Hard-very hard	30-90mins	200-300mins

These recommendations are consistent with the U.S. Department of Health & Human Services Physical Activity Guidelines for Americans.

Available for review at www.health.gov/PAGuidelines/pdf/paguide.pdf (U.S. Department of Health and Human Services, 2008) (ACSM, 2010, pp. 166-167).

Highlight and date the category you fall within and create your plan as indicated in the above sections. Before you even read the next chapter on Resistance Training, you must complete your exercise plan for cardiovascular activities as cardio is a stepping stone to resistance training. If you are extremely overweight and have never exercised before or you consider yourself a beginner exerciser, your first month of activity should contain only cardio focusing on LSD. Only after one month of cardio should you progress toward resistance training.

Popup Coach: The above content is extremely dense and rich with scientific facts about cardiovascular training and weight loss. View my video entitled, "Best Exercises to Burn Fat", to help decipher and create a cardio plan for yourself. https://www.youtube.com/watch?v=DkXvZdc4Ndc

CHAPTER 8

Resistance Training

Alas, the final component to creating and maintaining an effective weight loss plan is resistance training. Muscular fitness is an important component to maintaining a healthy lifestyle. Unfortunately, many people dislike and shy away from either the work it takes along with the resulting soreness, or they feel as though touching a weight will automatically transform their body into the Hulk or She-Hulk. Please allow me to clearly dispel this myth and impress upon you the value of resistance training. Your body is an amazing machine that was fearfully and wonderfully made, therefore it takes consistent work, effort and vigor to change anything about its current state. Your muscular system functions much like an elevator, if your desired location is the 13th floor, you must press the button associated with that floor. Do not be caught in the frenzy of people (this particularly happens in women) who are afraid to build muscle and shy away from the weight room. Skeletal muscle is created for the purpose of locomotion, and the lack of physical activity or movement in general, causes muscles to atrophy and decrease in ability. Not only is skeletal muscle a catalyst to movement, it is the substance that gives your body its beautiful shape and curves. Yes of course your bones set the structure, but you have the option of letting either muscle or fat fill in the outline.

The purpose of resistance training is to improve muscular fitness by increasing muscle strength, endurance and tone. The increase of strength can be accomplished without drastic increases in muscle size. There are trillions of muscle fibers in your body with varying sizes, each having a different maximal capacity for productivity. Increasing strength is increasing the ability of your muscles to function under various amounts of stress, and increases in endurance allow muscles to maintain high levels of stress for long periods of time. In order to look like a body builder, you must train like one with specific workouts catered towards muscle size which is different that training for strength or endurance. Though you may see similar exercises between yours and a body builder's routine, a body builder will train for mass with specific sets, reps and rest intervals which differ than those I will suggest later in this chapter. In other words, picking up a weight will not cause you to look like a body builder.

Without adequate muscle strength it becomes increasingly more difficult to perform daily tasks, and more difficult to perform high functioning activities. Your body will rise to the occasion of the tasks at hand, but injuries occur when the body is required to perform a task when it is not accustomed to functioning at such high levels.

Resistance training is an essential aspect to any physical fitness program and can take the form of weight lifting with free weights (dumbbells, plates, kettle bells), machine weights (stacked weights), resistance bands or even body weight activities where the resistance is your own weight fighting gravity. When creating a resistance training program for weight loss, it is important to create a plan with the focus of improving both muscular strength and endurance which will make the activities of daily living easier as well as effectively manage, attenuate and prevent the development of chronic diseases such as type 2 diabetes, osteoporosis, and obesity. For these vary reasons, resistance training increases in necessity as we age.

For the average individual seeking weight loss, resistance training should be performed 2-3 days per week (allowing for 48hrs rest in-between each session) with the focus on each major muscle group in each exercise session. The major muscle groups to focus on are chest, shoulders, upper and lower back, quadriceps, hamstrings, glutes, biceps, triceps and abdomen. I suggest training all major muscle groups in each exercise session allowing for a program that fosters total body growth. However, you may decide to focus on specific muscle groups on different days. Example; Quads, glutes, hams, biceps and shoulders on day one, Chest, upper back, lower back, triceps and calves on day two, or even choosing to focus on all upper body activities on one day and all lower body activities the next training session. There are many different ways to resistance train and many different patterns in which to do so, none of which are wrong, you just need to decide which works best for your schedule and which provides you with the best results.

How to Tame Your Body

After your cardiovascular warm up (regardless of whether your resistance exercise days are coupled with cardio, always do some type of cardio warm up for at least 5-10mins), you should prepare your body for the resistance training you are about to perform. This means performing light and simple variations of the muscle groups you plan to train as a means to properly prepare the body for resistance training. Example; if I am training chest, upper back and legs, I will begin my training session by not only stretching each of these muscle groups, but performing low intensity pushups (on the wall or floor depending on ability), deep body weight squats and shoulder roles. Dynamic warm up exercises, as those mentioned above, should always be performed in preparation for weight lifting.

Following the warm up, your order of exercises should follow this simple rule; organize your exercises by descending muscle size (step 1). Example, large muscles such as glutes, quads and chest should be the first exercises to complete on your exercise log. After arranging your exercises based upon muscle size, the next organizing criteria is the number of joints activated during the individual exercise selections. Therefore, exercises like squats will come before chest press due to squats working multiple large muscles (quads, glutes, and hams), and effecting multiple joint areas (ankles, knees, hips, spine, etc. – pretty much every joint in the body).

Remember, write your resistance training plan using the exercise log provided above (or create your own) in order of large muscle groups and max joint activations first, followed by smaller muscle groups and single joint activations. When completing your exercises in the weight room, also make sure to complete these activities for both sides of the body.

When engaging in resistance training there is one action that occurs in every repetition of activity composed of two opposing

> Stretching focuses on the muscle when it is in an eccentric state due to the purpose being to lengthen the muscle.

actions. A muscle contraction is the main action of resistance training but this full action has two associated categories called concentric and eccentric muscle actions. Concentric muscle actions occur anytime the muscle fibers are actively shortened. If I asked you to flex your bicep, you would raise your arm and contract your bicep by decreasing the distance between your forearm and bicep, therefore shortening the distance between your radius and ulna (forearm bones) and your humorous (the bone underneath the biceps). Concentric muscle contractions usually provide us with the muscle bulge or tone we wish to see. Eccentric muscle actions are the exact opposite. Eccentric muscle actions are muscle actions being lengthening under the stress of the shortening/concentric contraction. Flex your biceps again, now with your opposite hand, feel the tension of your triceps. Your triceps oppose the muscle action of the biceps when the biceps are flexing, just as your biceps oppose the muscle actions of the triceps when the triceps are flexing. This muscle opposition is how we maintain balance due to the constant battle of gaining control between primary and secondary muscles during every action. Additionally, every muscle has a concentric and eccentric action, the focus of the exercise dictates the stress of these actions. Remember, concentric is the shortening of muscle fibers while eccentric is the lengthening of muscle fibers. Example; the down phase of the squat is eccentric for the quads and upper hams, while the upward phase is concentric for the quads, upper hamstrings and glutes.

Your exercises should be focused on both concentric and eccentric action. Beware that the majority of muscle soreness comes from the eccentric phase. As the muscle lengthens under stress, some muscle fibers may be torn or stretched, causing microscopic inflammation that pushes on pain receptors. Individuals who are sore following exercise have experienced the above phenomena called DOMS (Delayed Onset Muscle Soreness). Stretching and a hot shower or bath will increase the blood flow to the effected muscles, washing away this excess inflammation. Don't be afraid of DOMS, embrace it! Feel the burn!

This Week's Design Your Body Fitness Challenge: Get Moving

I challenge you to exercise for at least one hour on 5 out of 7 days this week. Get up, get outside or hit the gym, but whatever you do... Just Get! I rarely do this but I think y'all are finally ready.

    I CHALLENGE you, I DARE you to try this workout plan for this week's challenge... BOOM!

Your Plan:
Monday: 20min hard run, 45mins hard weights (glutes, hams, quads, calf) abs
Tuesday: 30min run, 30 min weights (upper back, lower back, shoulders) abs
Wednesday: off, abs
Thursday: 40min hard cardio (game of hoops, swimming, biking, anything but running) 20min weights (biceps, triceps, lats) abs
Friday: 60 min hard weights (chest, low back, glutes, quads, hams, inner thigh, outer thigh)
Saturday: 60min cardio (exercise video, fitness class, play with the kids, elliptical, bball game etc.)
Sunday: off, abs

Post pics of your workouts on my page and show me how you get down!

Types of Resistance Training

There are three styles of resistance training; isotonic, isometric and isokinetic and our focus will be on the first two. As mentioned before, your body is a machine that needs to be fueled, lubricated and exercised. Just as there is optimal fuel types for your body, there are optimal resistance training activities you should participate in. Isotonic exercises refer to a constant force or tension applied to a muscle while the muscle's length changes. Every exercise goer consciously or unconsciously engages in isotonic exercises such as pushups, situps, pull ups, squats, biceps curls etc. Isotonic exercises are simply exercises that incorporate movement and have an up and/or down phase. Isometric exercises are those performed when the length of the muscle does not change. Isometric exercises include, but are not limited to: wall sits, planks, six-inches, pull up holds etc. Simply stated, Isotonic exercises are your dynamic (involve movement) exercises while isometrics incorporates static exercises.

Variation is key to creating and maintaining weight loss in your exercise plan. Incorporating changes in speed and count for the same exercise is an excellent way to vary intensity as you progress through your plan. Exercise variation and progression example: After two weeks of slow deep squats, incorporate a set of half-depth speed squats during weeks 3-4, then add jump squats weeks 5-8 while incorporating heavier and heavier weights on your jumps and watch your body change. Changing the speed of your exercise contractions is also important. The general rule of thumb for all resistance training is allowing two seconds for the contraction or up phase, and allowing four seconds for the eccentric or down phase. These times can be adjusted by either turning the isotonic exercise into an isometric exercise (no movement at all, you are just holding the exercise), or by increasing the speed at which each repetition is completed. Total repetitions performed is also a variation that will keep you mentally interested, and your body away from a plateau. If you begin your machine chest press exercise at 2 sets of 10 reps (2x10 is shorthand), during week 3-4, increase that number to 15 but do not sacrifice weight. If you increase your total number of reps, make sure your weights are increasing as well. In doing this you ensure that your body is performing optimally and that you are training for weight loss. Many people lose weight by cardio and endurance style resistance training only (high reps and low weight) but they are often extremely dissatisfied with the extra skin that has remained. Training for strength will increase muscle tone/size allowing your body to hold a good shape as it loses weight. I cannot guarantee that this will eradicate excess skin after weight loss but it certainly will cause you to be shapelier. The excess skin came from years of being stretched, it will take some time to conform to a new physique.

Below is a small matrix I have created for my readers. This chart is not extensive though it allows you to easily choose an exercise based upon the muscle group you desire to work. **Coach Cailah's Resistance Training Matrix** will greatly assist you in creating and updating your resistance training exercise log. In this log I have compiled the general exercise but I have not included the vast variations associated with each exercise.

There are hundreds of variations to exercises that will help keep you fresh and add progressions. Variations include moving from 2 arms/legs to single arm/leg activities, changing the surface from a stable surface to an instable surface (standing on a pillow, stabilizer ball etc.), changing your position of standing or sitting, or even changing direction (some exercises are performed in the vertical plane, why not move horizontally, diagonally or create your own circular motions?). Example, in the Free Weight Exercise column for the Chest muscle group, I only mention bench press and have not included its many variations such as incline bench press, decline bench press, or the various grips that change the way this exercise works and the number of muscle groups it innervates. I will allow you to explore the fun and creativity of creating your own plan and creating your own exercises.

Coach Cailah's Resistance Training Matrix

Exercise Matrix			
Muscle Group	**Machine**	**Free Weight**	**Body Weight**
Chest	Chest Press, Chest Fly	Bench press, Chest flys, Cable cross over	Pushups, (Close grip, Wide grip or neutral), Dips
Biceps	Arm curl	DB curl, Preacher curl, Hammer curl	Chin ups
Triceps	Triceps push down/extensions,	Triceps kick back, Overhead triceps extensions, Close grip bench press, close grip pull downs	Dips, Pull ups, Close grip push ups
Deltoids (anterior, middle and posterior)	Shoulder press, Shoulder side raise, Low row, Chest Press	Bench press, Front and Side DB raises, and anything overhead, Shoulder press	Pull ups, Chin ups, pushups, Dips
Abdominals	Abdominal crunch, Abdominal twist	Planks, Crunches, Situps Bicycles, Twists, Any movement crunching your shoulders towards your hips or knees (or vice versa), includes twisting and other patterns, or isometric actions both while holding weight	Planks, Crunches, Situps, Bicycles, Twists, Any movement crunching your shoulders towards your hips or knees (or vice versa) includes twisting and other patterns, or isometric actions
Obliques (Internal/External)	Abdominal twist	DB Oblique crunches, any pulling activity that requires rotation, Diagonal chops, side planks	Standing oblique crunches, Side planks, any rotational action where the opposing sides of your body meet (right hand and left foot)
Gluteus Maximus	Leg press, Leg sled, Hack squat, Glute kick back	Squats, Lunges, anything involving a deep jump, Dead lifts	Squats, lunges, anything involving a deep jump
Quadriceps	Leg press, Leg sled, Hack squat, Glute kick back, Leg extension	Squats, Lunges, anything involving a deep jump, Dead lifts	Squats, lunges, anything involving a deep jump, Front kicking
Hamstrings	Leg press, Leg sled, Hack squat, Glute kick back, Leg curl	Squats, Lunges, anything involving a deep jump, Dead lifts, Straight leg dead lifts	Squats, lunges, anything involving a deep jump, lying bent knee hip thrusts
Calves	Standing or seated Calf raise machine, these activities can be performed on any leg press	Standing or seated calf raise, anything jumping	Standing calf raise, anything jumping
Forearms	NA	Weighted wrist rolls, DB wrist curls, Grip trainers	Fingertip pushups, manual resistance wrist manipulation
Latissumus Dorsi (Lats)	Lat pulldown, High row,	Cable cross over/pull down	Wide grip pull up, Lat Push Up
Trapezius (Traps/upper back)	High row, Low row	Shoulder shrug, Shoulder front and side raise, Cable cross over pulls, Close grip pull downs	Shoulder pushups, Pull ups, Chin ups, Dips
Erector Spinae	Back extension	Hyperextension chair, Supermans, Squats, Dead lifts, anything overhead	Supermans
Adductors (inner thigh)	Adductor machine	Cable machine medial leg swings	Laying medial leg raise, exercise ball squeezes
Abductors (outter thigh)	Abductor machine	Cable machine lateral leg swings, Lateral lunges, Skiiers, Lateral hops, anything with a reversable lateral motion	Lateral lunges, Skiiers, Lateral hops, anything with a reversable lateral motion

Volume and Training for Weight Loss

When exercising, each muscle group should be worked 2-4 times during each training session. Example, you can perform four sets of squats (active muscles are glutes, quads and hams) at 10 reps each or perform two sets of squats and two sets of leg extensions (quads) followed by two sets of leg curls (hams). This method of using different exercises to work the same muscle groups add variety to your training program and it decreases the potential for staleness (ACSM, 2010, p. 169). Following each set your goal should be a rest interval of 30-90s. It is extremely important to plan your rest time. Each time you enter the gym you should have a watch or clock to time your timed exercises as well as your rest. A rest period of 30-90s in between each exercise is optimal along with a rest period of 1-2 minutes in between each new exercise set. Timing your rest intervals appropriately aid your body in weight loss due to various physiological and chemical properties.

Referring back to the FITT (Frequency, Intensity, Time and Type) framework, the number of repetitions and level of intensity is inversely related. This means that the lower number of repetitions and the higher amount of weight used reflects a higher intensity, just as the higher number of repetitions and the lower weight used indicates lower activity exercises. As stated above, your goal should be to stay within the middle of this continuum. Repetitions of 8-12 and at times, 20, are adequate repetition counts for weight loss. Begin with 3-4 sets of 12 reps of each exercise. But you must remember that your weight should increase as your exercises continue. Challenge yourself.

How can you tell what weight is appropriate for the number of repetitions you chose? Simple, the most important indicator of resistance training intensity is how difficult it is to complete the last repetition. If it is extremely easy for you to complete rep 12 out of a 12 repetition set, this means the weight is too light and you need to increase resistance. You should be struggling to complete the last rep of each set. This is a good indicator that your muscles are working at a high enough capacity to induce change. Equally as important, if your muscles fail to complete the full 12 repetition set, you need to reduce the weight and mark all changes in your exercise log. This means that breathing and grunting may be necessary (plus it's fun to do)! Control your breathing during your resistance training (exhale on exertion).You must put forth continual effort in your resistance training during your weight loss journey.

Below is a three week plan you can use, combined with **Coach Cailah's Resistance Training Matrix,** to create your own exercise plan. My suggestion is first set your resistance training frequency (2-3d/wk), then fill in the below exercise log with the different exercises and muscle groups you will work each day. After completing three weeks of 2-3 days of resistance training, follow the progression guidelines for creating another exercise plan, or simply modifying the existing plan by increasing the intensity (this scan be done by increasing sets, reps and/or weight).

It is important to incorporate proper rest as a part of your exercise plan. This rest should be active where you participate in physical activity style exercises or low/no impact days. Every 3 weeks of consistent training, I suggest you build into your schedule a few low intensity days to refresh your mind and to give your body a quick break. The most amount of time you should take off from exercise is 1 week, but this card should be cashed in sparingly. Remember, you should enjoy this process, if you don't, you won't stick to it.

Cailah's Sample Weight Lifting Chart

	Date:			Date:			Date:		
Exercise	Sets	Reps	Weight	Sets	Reps	Weight	Sets	Reps	Weight

Returning to Exercise after a Break

There will be times throughout your journey where you may fall off track and you will need to reassess and rewrite your workout schedule. If, and when, this happens, depending upon how long you've been inactive, you should not begin your exercise plan where you left off. Science proves that after three days of inactivity, your muscles begin to atrophy. Though you may not physically see these changes, your body loses muscle mass, organic makeup (mitochondria and various enzymes) and therefore performance levels decrease. Taking a week off for the purpose of active rest during your active training schedule is important and after a week of inactivity, you do not need to rewrite your exercise plan and may resume where you left. If this break or stent of inactivity last for two to three weeks, decrease your intensity and exercise times in order to recalibrate your body.

Remember, varying your intensity is accomplished by varying weight used, speed of activity, sets, repetitions, and associated distances. Most people have the ability to maintain exercise frequency (days/week) after a 2-3 week stent away from exercise, but only when total intensity is decreased. Total exercise time also needs to decrease. Though intensity and exercise time need to change, if you are returning from inactivity within three weeks, you may resume your exercise plan with the noted adjustments above. If you are returning to exercise from longer than a 1-month break, you need to completely restructure your exercise plan. Review the FITT framework and adjust each exercise as necessary. Upon returning to exercise Frequency, Intensity and Time should all drastically decrease.

These breaks will happen throughout your lifestyle change, do not let them discourage you, just reassess, adjust and get back on the ball!

"Stay on the path, fight through the struggle, and you will find success."
-Cailah Brock

I Only Have 10 Minutes

You may not always have 1hr to dedicate to your workout regimen, but that should not discourage you from working out. If time is limited your goal should be completing exercises that require large muscle groups, multiple joints, and full body movements at high intensities in the least amount of time. Circuit and HIIT (High Intensity Interval Training) are typically the best options to utilize given this setting. As stated above, circuit training is a system of training that requires multiple types of exercises be revisited within a set time period and with little rest. High Intensity Interval Training (HIIT) is very similar but only incorporates high intensity exercises.

When creating a circuit training workout, choose 3-7 exercises (this group of exercises is called a set or circuit) that collectively address each muscle group. Exercise options can range from hill runs to pushups, there is no limitation. Adding a circuit training day to your workout will not only burn high amounts of calories, but it will keep your workouts fresh. The goal of circuit training is to complete a specific number of sets or rounds base on the level of intensity and in order to do so, you must set exercise parameters.

Here are a few things to keep in mind when creating your workout;

- **What is my exercise duration?** This is not referring to the total time it takes you to complete the workout, but this reflects the unit of measurement to use in order to indicate when you have completed an exercise in your set/circuit. This measurement can be set by time or repetition dependencies. Example, you can do 50 jumping jacks or do jumping jacks for 60s before moving to the next exercise.
- **How many circuits or sets for the entire workout?** This should be dependent on your fitness level and the duration of each exercise. Generally, begin by completing 1-2 sets of 3-4 exercises

to test your fitness level, then adjust your intensity by adding sets, reps or extending your exercise duration.

- **Indicate a rest interval.** After you complete each set/round, there should be a set time for rest. Do not allow your rest to be an arbitrary figure but set the specific time just as you would set times for sets and reps.

Example circuit training workout that only takes 10-15mins to complete:

20 push ups

60s of jumping jacks

15 squat jumps

60s high knees

30s defensive slides

2-3 minute rest

Complete 3-4 sets

Pop Up Coach: Check out this exercise video entitled, "10min Full Body Workout" **https://www.youtube.com/watch?v=9v6HxJU4ZXU**

The Secret to a Flat Stomach

The illustrious flat stomach; health seekers want it, fitness gurus have it, and your question is how to get it. It is true, some people are naturally skinny or small and it is easier for them to maintain their idea of a "fit" body. Some gain muscle faster than others while others gain fat within the blink of an eye. So yes, genetics does play a role in the adaptations of your body, and also be realistic with yourself and know that your body does have limitations. My first and only warning to you comes as an announcement and a plea. Please do not compare yourself to someone else, especially the unrealistic body types we see on television. I encourage you to love yourself through each stage of your change. Still set your goal, but do not compare yourself to another, be satisfied from within.

The trick to acquiring and maintaining a flat stomach comes with balancing the Trinity of Health and Wellness. You must have an adequate nutrition, along with a good calorie burning cardio regimen and of course, a total body resistance training program. In order to have a flat stomach you must lose fat and build muscle equally. If you only lose fat, your stomach will be small but have no shape and still be loose and you will see no definition or curve. If you only build muscle, you will have a solid midsection but still, no definition or curve. If you have entered this race while in the beginning phases of your health seeking journey and one of your goals is to have a flat stomach, I encourage you to focus on total body calorie burn with both cardio and resistance training. Remember, spot training does not work, but also remember the SAID Principle states that your body will adapt to stressors. The secret to a flat stomach is participating in whole body, high calorie burning cardio and resistance training while putting an extra emphasis on the abdominal section and participating in multiple types of trunk (midsection or core) building activities. If your abs are not appropriately stressed you will not see results. This means that when you do abs exercises, consider adding weight as you progress in fitness level.

Though we call them "Abs", your stomach is composed of more muscles than simply your Rectus Abdominis, the prized muscle that produces the coveted six-pack. There are five major muscles that will help sculpt and define your midsection; Rectus Abdominis, Internal and External Obliques, Transvers Abdominis and a group of muscles known as the Erector Spinae. Each muscle can be activated by different exercises and it is important to make sure your routine hits each muscle group.

Below is a quick guide discussing how to activate each of the major muscles within the trunk:

- **Rectus Abdominis:** Any crunching movement where you decrease the angle between your shoulders and hips activates the rectus abdominis. This muscle is activated by any linear crunching movement.

- **Internal and External Obliques:** Technically two different muscles, the internal and external obliques which are activated when participating in diagonal trunk exercises due to the orientation of the muscle fibers. These muscles are also activated when performing lateral movements that involve bending laterally at the waist.

- **Transverse Abdominis:** Known as your "corset" muscle, the transverse abdominis is purposed to protect internal organs and keep them in place. Twisting motions will activate this muscle.

- **Erector Spinae:** One of the many muscle groups of the back, the erector spinae group helps your body stay erect and stand straight. Many people forget to exercise their lower back as frequently and with the same intensity as they do their abs, and are oblivious to the issues this particular muscle imbalance can cause. This muscle group is activated by any exercise that increases the angle at the hips against resistance.

Each of these muscles will contract and operate during a large majority of ab exercises you choose. Still, be mindful of the different muscles in this area and choose exercises that will produce the best results for each of these muscle groups.

At this point, take a full body photo (front, side and back) and mark this date as your "after" or "midway" photo: Date: _____. Submit to this photo to me detailing your exercise journey and the results this book has allowed you to reach.

THE RE-EVALUATION

Here is an excellent time to reevaluate your physiological condition. If you have dropped more than 15lbs or 5% of your body weight, revisit the charts back in the section titled 'Determining Your Risk Factors' and see how you have progressed. I also encourage you to schedule a doctor's appointment and ask them to reevaluate you (including blood work) as your goal is to decrease the amount or dosage of medication you are taking.

Based on the CVD (cardiovascular disease) charts for signs and symptoms, and risk factors, I now categorized as (circle one):

    a.   Low Risk and I can begin exercise immediately.

          a.   I've not been diagnosed with a CVD, nor do I have any signs or symptoms of a CVD and I have < 2 risk factors.

    b.   Moderate Risk and I can engage in low to moderate intensity exercise (40-60% of maximal effort).

          a.   I've not been diagnosed with a CVD, nor do I have any signs or symptoms of a CVD but I have ≥ 2 risk factors.

    c.   High Risk and I should consult a physician to receive a medical examination and clearance before I begin my physical activity.

          a.   I have ≥ 1 sign or symptom of a CVD, and/or I have been diagnosed with a CVD, pulmonary and/or metabolic disease. This category is not dependent upon risk factors as the signs or symptoms are indicators of disease.

Revisit the Trinity Figures Scale in Chapter 4

Nutrition: _____   Cardiovascular Endurance_____   Resistance Training_____
      Date: _____   Current Weight: _____

CHAPTER 9

Things That Can Sabotage Your Weight Loss

Though you now have the tools to create an effective weight loss plan, you need to prepare yourself for the reality that certain obstacles may fall directly in your path to success. You may weigh yourself and get discouraged due to weight fluctuations or even weight gain. Be encouraged. For some people, weight loss is more than mastering the ration of calories in to calories out, some may have extra challenges that hinder them from their desired weight loss.

Food Sensitivities:

Certain foods you consume may cause adverse reactions in your body that are too mild to be considered allergic reactions, though they may affect your ability to lose weight. Just as childhood obesity may be linked with food allergies, these same food allergies may stay with you throughout adulthood. As you are aware, not all food allergens are life threatening and eating foods that your body may be intolerant to may cause water retention or even inflammation. Food cravings may also affect your health. According to Pamela Wartian Smith, M.D., subtle intolerances to various foods cause an increase in epinephrine which literally gives your body a "high", causing you to be physically drawn to particular foods which are not always healthy. The solution to this issue can be easier said than done. Track and eliminate the foods you are overly sensitive to in your diet.

Inconsistencies:

Inconsistency is a killer of dreams. As committed as you were to reach your weight loss goals when beginning this book, as you finish it, you should remain as committed; and I would not be surprised if you found an increased level of enthusiasm about gaining and maintaining your weight loss. Stay on track, stay the course, stay consistently committed and you will succeed. The only failure is quitting when you have gone so far in your journey. DO NOT allow your schedule to grab hold of your health, fight to make the time to meal prep, eat right and exercise. Fight to make time to maintain your life.

Stress Levels:

High levels of stress can increase your "fight or flight" hormone (cortisol) response which can break down muscle fibers, impair glucose/ blood sugar metabolism and increase food cravings. Also, losing 1 hour of sleep for 3 nights can also cause an adverse reaction which increases the appetite and suppresses the chemical releases that tell your body you are full (Institute of Medicine, 1995).

Thyroid Gland Issues:

The purpose of the thyroid gland is to regulate the rate of metabolism, therefore, weight loss and weight gain. Improperly functioning thyroids can cause weight gain and many other medical complications. Nearly 1/3rd of all Americans have a thyroid that is operating at suboptimal levels which can be brought about from genetics, stress and/or sleep deprivation. There is also science indicating that those who consistently eat too few calories (less than 1,700cals for women and 2,000cals for men), and those who consistently participate in vigorous exercise more than 90mins/day are more likely to have thyroid gland issues. If you have issues with this gland (over or underactivity) consult your physician for best courses of action.

Personal Battles:

Each of us have an internal struggle with obstacles and situations that can halt our progress and even deter us from ever beginning. Before discussing the pain, time commitment, discomfort, struggles in finding facilities, lack of support, injuries and other external factors, many times the most challenging issues that need overcoming are generated from within. Personally, I still face struggles in my workout and in maintaining faithfulness to good nutrition. Some may simply say, "Just exercise self-control", when many times the fight must begin with gaining control of what drives you. Example, I do not enjoy running; I actually hate it. This may come as a surprise to some of you, but running is neither my strongest, nor favorite component of exercising as it is long and boring. However, because I understand running to be one of the most beneficial and fastest ways to burn large amounts of calories with minimal equipment, I have incorporated this activity into my workout regimen. Almost every time I run, my mind tells me to stop, to slow down, to walk at the next corner, to sandbag the curve or to sometimes, turn around and go home! Not only is running hard enough, but now I must battle my mind for control of my actions and therefore success.

Your mind is an extremely powerful and persuasive tool that either fights alongside you or against you. For some, gaining control of your mind is considered enlightenment. For the rest of us who have yet to reach that level, note that you will enter into frequent battles with your mind. In these situations, the question becomes, who will win? At times, your mind will not stop churning and producing thoughts, but as long as your activity does not decline, you win. Do not give in to external or internal occurrences that will hinder your progress. Fight the world to acquire and maintain control of yourself, and to lead you to success.

You will win only when you enter the ring to challenge the obstacle. Realize that many times, that obstacle can be "You". Fight yourself, be a contender, control your mind and control your actions. As long as you enter the ring, you win. You may not win each battle, but at least enter the ring each day and create the opportunity to move yourself into an environment that breaths success, triumph and accomplishment.

"...Success is failure turned inside out...,
It might be near when it seems afar;
So stick to the fight when you're hardest hit,
It's when things seem worst that you must not quit."
- Edgar A. Guest, an excerpt from the poem "Don't Quit"

Self-Doubt:

"Doubt sees the obstacle, faith sees the way, doubt sees the darkest
night, faith sees the day, doubt dreads to take a step, faith soars
on high, doubt questions, "who believes?", faith answers, "I!""
-William (Harvey) Jett, "Doubt vs. Faith"

Self-doubt is the single most dangerous influence in your life. You control your mind just as you control your body. It takes an active as well as continuous effort to undo every unhealthy thing your body has had to endure over the past years. Refer back to your goals continuously as a reminder for what your hard work is for and what you wish to accomplish. Also reward yourself for reaching benchmarks. Through this process, don't be afraid to live your life. Don't restrict yourself from good living, just change what you view as good. A night out on the town after dinner is an excellent way to blow off steam, burn calories and enjoy yourself. Don't forget to enjoy life, this is a process to improving you, enjoy the ride. Believe in yourself! You are great, you are beautiful, you are improving you.

"The continuous improvement of you"
-Kenton Davis

WORKS CITED

ACE - American Council on Exercise. (2011). *ACE Lifestyle and Weight Management Coach Manual* (Vol. 2). (C. X. Bryant, Ed.) San Diego, CA: American Council on Exercise.

ACSM. (2010). Preparticipation Health Screening and Risk Stratification. In A. C. Medicine, *ACSM's Guidelines for Exercise Testing and Prescription* (p. 380). Baltimore: Wolters Kluwer.

Austrailian Bureau of Statistics/Commonwealth Department of Health and Ageing. (1998). *Protein*. Retrieved from Nutrient Reference Values for Austrailia and New Zeland: http://www.nrv.gov.au/nutrients/protein

Bizla. (2012, November 14). *RIGGED Obese Man Base Model*. Retrieved from Turbo Squid: http://www.turbosquid.com/3d-models/3d-model-rigged-base-mesh/706389

Brown, A. (2004). *Understanding Food: Principles and Preparation* (Vol. 2). (E. Howe, Ed.) Belmont, California: Wadsworth/Thomson Learning.

Bryant, C. X., & Green, D. J. (2011). *ACE Lifestyle & Weight Management Coach manual.* San Diego, CA 92123: American Council on Exercise.

Exercise, T. A. (2013). Numbers to Know Body Mass Index. *Fit Facts.* San Diego. Retrieved from acefit.com_BMI_Calculator

ExRx.net. (2014, March 16). *Diet and Nutrition*. Retrieved from Exercise Prescription: http://www.exrx.net/Nutrition.html

Hinckley, D. (2012, September 19). *Entertainment*. Retrieved from New York Daily News: http://www.nydailynews.com/entertainment/

tv-movies/americans-spend-34-hours-week-watching-tv-nielsen-numbers-article-1.1162285

Hinckley, D. (2014, March 5). *Entertainment*. Retrieved from New York Daily News: http://www.nydailynews.com/life-style/average-american-watches-5-hours-tv-day-article-1.1711954

Institute of Medicine. (1995). *Weighing the Options: Criteria for Evaluating Weight-Management Programs*. Washington, D.C.: National Academy Press.

Nelson, R.D., L.D., J. K. (2012, September 27). *Nutrition and Healthy Living*. Retrieved from Mayo Clinic: http://www.mayoclinic.org/healthy-living/nutrition-and-healthy-eating/expert-answers/high-fructose-corn-syrup/faq-20058201

Prochaska, J., & Marcus, B. (1994). The transtheoretical model; Apllications to exercise. *Advances in Exercise Adherence*.

Skov, A. R., Toubro, S., Holm, L., & Astrup, A. (1999). Randomized trial on protein vs carbohydrate in adlibitum fat reduced for the treatment of obesity. *International Journal of Obesity Relaated Metabolic Disorders, 23*(5), 528-36.

The American Council on Exercise. (2013). *Fit Facts*. (The American Council on Exercise) Retrieved from Knowing Your Numbers: Body Mass Index: http://www.acefitness.org/fitness-fact-article/3594/know-your-numbers-body-mass-index/

U.S. Department of Health and Human Services. (2008). *Physical Activity Guidelines for Americans*. Retrieved from Physical Activity Guidelines: www.health.gov/PAGuidelines/pdf/paguide.pdf